T0263335

The Diabetic Charcot Foot and Ankle: A Multidisciplinary Team Approach

Editor

THOMAS ZGONIS

CLINICS IN PODIATRIC MEDICINE AND SURGERY

www.podiatric.theclinics.com

Consulting Editor
THOMAS ZGONIS

January 2017 • Volume 34 • Number 1

ELSEVIER

1600 John F. Kennedy Boulevard • Suite 1800 • Philadelphia, Pennsylvania, 19103-2899

http://www.theclinics.com

CLINICS IN PODIATRIC MEDICINE AND SURGERY Volume 34, Number 1
January 2017 ISSN 0891-8422, ISBN-13: 978-0-323-48269-1

Editor: Jennifer Flynn-Briggs
Developmental Editor: Alison Swety

Clinics in Podiatric Medicine and Surgery (ISSN 0891-8422) is published quarterly by Elsevier Inc., 360 Park Avenue South, New York, NY 10010-1710. Months of issue are January, April, July, and October. Business and Editorial Offices: 1600 John F. Kennedy Blvd., Ste. 1800, Philadelphia, PA 19103-2899. Customer Service Office: 3251 Riverport Lane, Maryland Heights, MO 63043. Periodicals postage paid at New York, NY and additional mailing offices. Subscription prices are $288.00 per year for US individuals, $518.00 per year for US institutions, $100.00 per year for US students and residents, $374.00 per year for Canadian individuals, $626.00 for Canadian institutions, $439.00 for international individuals, $626.00 per year for international institutions and $220.00 per year for Canadian and foreign students/residents. To receive student/resident rate, orders must be accompanied by name of affiliated institution, date of term, and the *signature* of program/residency coordinator on institution letterhead. Orders will be billed at individual rate until proof of status is received. Foreign air speed delivery is included in all *Clinics* subscription prices. All prices are subject to change without notice. POSTMASTER: Send address changes to *Clinics in Podiatric Medicine and Surgery*, Elsevier Health Sciences Division, Subscription Customer Service, 3251 Riverport Lane, Maryland Heights, MO 63043. **Customer Service: 1-800-654-2452 (US). From outside of the US, call 314-447-8871. Fax: 314-447-8029. E-mail: JournalsCustomerService-usa@elsevier.com (for print support); JournalsOnlineSupport-usa@elsevier.com (for online support).**

Reprints. For copies of 100 or more of articles in this publication, please contact the Commercial Reprints Department, Elsevier Inc., 360 Park Avenue South, New York, NY 10010-1710. Tel.: 212-633-3874; Fax: 212-633-3820; E-mail: reprints@elsevier.com.

Clinics in Podiatric Medicine and Surgery is covered in *MEDLINE/PubMed (Index Medicus) and EMBASE/Excerpta Medica.*

CLINICS IN PODIATRIC MEDICINE AND SURGERY

Contributors

CONSULTING EDITOR

THOMAS ZGONIS, DPM, FACFAS
Professor and Director, Externship and Reconstructive Foot and Ankle Fellowship Programs, Division of Podiatric Medicine and Surgery, Department of Orthopaedics, University of Texas Health Science Center San Antonio, San Antonio, Texas

EDITOR

THOMAS ZGONIS, DPM, FACFAS
Professor and Director, Externship and Reconstructive Foot and Ankle Fellowship Programs, Division of Podiatric Medicine and Surgery, Department of Orthopaedics, University of Texas Health Science Center San Antonio, San Antonio, Texas

AUTHORS

YOUSEF ALRASHIDI, MD
Assistant Professor, Orthopaedic Department, Orthopaedic Foot and Ankle Surgeon, College of Medicine, Taibah University, Almadinah Almunawwarah, Kingdom of Saudi Arabia; Clinical Fellow, Orthopaedic Department, Schmerzklinik Basel, Swiss Medical Network, Basel, Switzerland

PATRICK R. BURNS, DPM
Assistant Professor of Orthopaedic Surgery, University of Pittsburgh School of Medicine; Director, UPMC Podiatric Medicine and Surgery Residency, Pittsburgh, Pennsylvania

CLAIRE M. CAPOBIANCO, DPM, FACFAS
Attending, Orthopaedic Associates of Southern Delaware, Lewes, Delaware

MICHAEL E. EDMONDS, MD, FRCP
Diabetic Foot Clinic, King's College Hospital NHS Foundation Trust, London, United Kingdom

THOMAS HÜGLE, MD, PhD
Assistant Professor and Head, Rheumatology Department, Osteoarthritis Research Center Basel, Schmerzklinik Basel, Swiss Medical Network, Basel, Switzerland

MARIO HERRERA-PEREZ, MD
Assistant Professor of Orthopaedics, Universidad de La Laguna, University Hospital of Canary Islands, Tenerife, Spain

SPENCER J. MONACO, DPM
PGY-3, UPMC Podiatric Medicine and Surgery Residency, Pittsburgh, Pennsylvania

TAHIR ÖGÜT, MD
Professor, Department of Orthopaedics and Traumatology, Cerrahpasa Medical School, Istanbul University, Istanbul, Turkey

NINA L. PETROVA, MD, PhD
Diabetic Foot Clinic, King's College Hospital NHS Foundation Trust, London, United Kingdom

CRYSTAL L. RAMANUJAM, DPM, MSc
Assistant Professor/Clinical, Division of Podiatric Medicine and Surgery, Department of Orthopaedics, University of Texas Health Science Center San Antonio, San Antonio, Texas

DANIEL J. SHORT, DPM
Specialist and Fellow, Reconstructive Foot and Ankle Surgery, Division of Podiatric Medicine and Surgery, Department of Orthopaedics, University of Texas Health Science Center San Antonio, San Antonio, Texas

VICTOR VALDERRABANO, MD, PhD
Professor and Head, Orthopaedic Department, Osteoarthritis Research Center Basel, Schmerzklinik Basel, Swiss Medical Network, Basel, Switzerland

MARTIN WIEWIORSKI, MD
Consultant, Chief of the Foot and Ankle Section, Department of Orthopaedic Surgery and Traumatology, Kantonsspital Winterthur, Winterthur, Switzerland

NECIP SELCUK YONTAR, MD
Faculty, Department of Orthopaedics and Traumatology, Istanbul Cerrahi Hospital, Istanbul, Turkey

THOMAS ZGONIS, DPM, FACFAS
Professor and Director, Externship and Reconstructive Foot and Ankle Fellowship Programs, Division of Podiatric Medicine and Surgery, Department of Orthopaedics, University of Texas Health Science Center San Antonio, San Antonio, Texas

Contents

prognosis. Its surgical management is equally difficult to interpret based on the wide array of options available. In the presence of an ulceration or concomitant osteomyelitis, internal fixation by means of screws, plates, or intramedullary nailing needs to be avoided when feasible. External fixation becomes a great surgical tool when managing DCN with concomitant osteomyelitis. This article describes internal and external fixation methods along with available literature to enlighten surgeons faced with treating this complex condition.

Surgical Equinus Correction for the Diabetic Charcot Foot: What the Evidence Reveals **33**

Claire M. Capobianco

Triceps surae contracture, or equinus, is a known deforming force in the foot and ankle. Biomechanical studies have shown that ankle equinus significantly alters gait and plantar pressures, and in the diabetic neuropathic patient population, this can propagate plantar ulceration and/or Charcot neuroarthropathy (CN). Surgical correction of equinus is globally and frequently used to aid in plantar wound healing in the neuropathic diabetic patient, with and without CN. Treatment guidelines for equinus correction in this medically complex population are undefined and lack evidence from high-quality published peer-reviewed studies.

Surgical Treatment Options for the Diabetic Charcot Midfoot Deformity **43**

Yousef Alrashidi, Thomas Hügle, Martin Wiewiorski, Mario Herrera-Perez, and Victor Valderrabano

Management of diabetic Charcot midfoot deformity is one of the most demanding aspects of foot and ankle surgery. Its treatment should aim at reducing the rate of complications, including foot and ankle amputations or limb loss. Attempting reconstruction at Eichenholtz stages I and II carries the risk of infection and loss of fixation. It is advisable to limit surgical reconstruction to Eichenholtz stage III in the absence of any evidence of infection or vascular insufficiency. Achilles lengthening or gastrocnemius-soleus release is an essential initial step in surgery. Addressing the medial foot column first is a key to a successful reconstruction.

Surgical Treatment Options for the Diabetic Charcot Hindfoot and Ankle Deformity **53**

Tahir Ögüt and Necip Selcuk Yontar

Charcot neuroarthropathy is associated with progressive, noninfectious, osteolysis-induced bone and joint destruction. When the ankle and/or hindfoot is affected by the destruction process, management is further complicated with collapse and destruction of the talar body, which increases instability around the ankle. In this patient population, arthrodesis is the most commonly used surgical procedure. Internal fixation, external fixation, or a combination of both can be used for the treatment. Decision making between them should be individualized according to the patient characteristics.

Soft Tissue Reconstruction Pyramid for the Diabetic Charcot Foot 69

Claire M. Capobianco and Thomas Zgonis

Foot and ankle ulcerations in patients with diabetic Charcot neuroarthropathy (DCN) occur frequently and can be challenging to address surgically when conservative care fails. Patients with acute or chronic diabetic foot ulcers (DFU) are at continued risk for development of osteomyelitis, septic arthritis, gas gangrene, and potential lower extremity amputation. Concurrent vasculopathy and peripheral neuropathy as well as uncontrolled medical comorbidities complicate the treatment approach. In addition, pathomechanical forces left untreated may contribute to DFU recurrence in this patient population. This article outlines in detail the stepwise approach and options available for durable soft tissue coverage in the DCN patient.

Revisional Surgery of the Diabetic Charcot Foot and Ankle 77

Patrick R. Burns and Spencer J. Monaco

Charcot neuroarthropathy (CN) is a difficult problem for the foot and ankle surgeon. If surgery is required, little is known or available regarding the best methods and timing. When the initial attempt of reconstruction fails, revision of CN is even more demanding. One must take in to account all aspects, including nutrition, vascular status, infection control, short- and long-term blood glucose management, as well as other factors requiring laboratory monitoring and consult services. Once optimized, the biomechanics of the deformity can be addressed and decisions can be made on fixation devices.

Circular External Fixation as a Primary or Adjunctive Therapy for the Podoplastic Approach of the Diabetic Charcot Foot 93

Daniel J. Short and Thomas Zgonis

Numerous techniques have been described for surgical management of the diabetic Charcot foot. External fixation has become a main surgical tool for the reconstructive foot and ankle surgeon when dealing with the ulcerated diabetic Charcot foot. In the presence of an open wound and/or osteomyelitis, staged reconstruction with circular external fixation becomes ideal for salvage of the diabetic lower extremity. Also, circular external fixation can provide simultaneous compression and stabilization, correct the underlying osseous or soft tissue deformities, and surgically offload the diabetic Charcot foot. This article describes a variety of circular external fixation applications for the diabetic Charcot foot.

Index 99

CLINICS IN PODIATRIC MEDICINE AND SURGERY

Preface

The Diabetic Charcot Foot and Ankle: A Multidisciplinary Team Approach

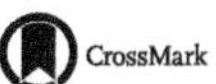

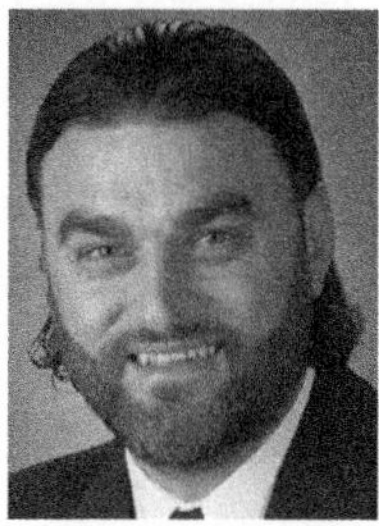

Thomas Zgonis, DPM, FACFAS
Editor

I am honored and humbled to serve as a guest editor for this *Clinics in Podiatric Medicine and Surgery* issue focused on the diagnosis and management of the diabetic Charcot foot and ankle. Knowledge of diagnosing and treating the diabetic Charcot foot and/or ankle has grown tremendously since the pathology was first described in a diabetic patient by William Riely Jordan in 1936. For the last 80 years, conservative and surgical treatments have been well advanced based on technological improvements, including but not limited to bracing, bone stimulation, drug administration, and surgical fixation methods of internal, external, or combined systems. However, even though there is a plethora of surgical techniques and instrumentation to address this rare but devastating surgical entity, little is known about its true pathophysiology and prevention in the diabetic population.

The literature since Jean-Martin Charcot's findings in 1868 has been fulfilled with many misdiagnoses and nomenclatures associated with the patient's condition and pathology. The diabetic patient with dense peripheral neuropathy and Charcot joint(s) represents a subspecialty diabetic group population that may differ in the diagnosis and treatment seen in Charcot neuroarthropathy patients due to chronic alcoholism, congenital or chronic insensitivity to pain, leprosy, peripheral nerve lesions, idiopathic neuropathy, and others. The diagnosis and treatment of the diabetic Charcot foot can be quite challenging in the presence of open wounds and osteomyelitis. Furthermore, the surgical reconstruction of the diabetic Charcot foot faces bigger challenges in the presence of hyperglycemia, vasculopathy, nephropathy, neuropathy, concomitant osteomyelitis, cardiac disease, and decreased bone mineral density. Understanding the cause and pathophysiology of the "diabetic Charcot-Jordan foot" as well as establishing a unifying consensus on the accurate nomenclature, classification, treatment strategies, and preventive measures through a diabetic multidisciplinary team

Clin Podiatr Med Surg 34 (2017) xi–xii
http://dx.doi.org/10.1016/j.cpm.2016.10.001
0891-8422/17/© 2016 Published by Elsevier Inc.

approach will lead to future research and registry data collection of successfully treating this complex and devastating condition.

In this issue, the national and international invited authors have done an excellent job in covering the diagnosis and treatment of the diabetic Charcot foot and ankle. Various topics from medical imaging to pharmacologic therapy and surgical reconstruction are described in detail that can be used as a great reference to our readers. In conclusion, I personally would like to thank all of the guest editors, invited authors, editorial board members, editorial staff at Elsevier, and our readers for their outstanding contributions and input in the *Clinics in Podiatric Medicine and Surgery.*

Thomas Zgonis, DPM, FACFAS
Externship and Reconstructive Foot and
Ankle Fellowship Programs
Division of Podiatric Medicine and Surgery
Department of Orthopaedics
University of Texas Health
Science Center San Antonio
7703 Floyd Curl Drive-MSC 7776
San Antonio, TX 78229, USA

E-mail address:
zgonis@uthscsa.edu

The Diabetic Charcot Foot from 1936 to 2016

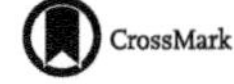

Eighty Years Later and Still Growing

Crystal L. Ramanujam, DPM, MSc, Thomas Zgonis, DPM*

KEYWORDS

- Diabetic Charcot foot • Charcot neuroarthropathy • Diabetic Charcot-Jordan Foot • Diabetic neuropathy • Charcot classification • Diabetes mellitus

KEY POINTS

- Much of the literature surrounding diabetic Charcot neuroarthropathy (DCN) since its first description in 1936 has focused on advances in diagnosis and treatment.
- A multidisciplinary approach is encouraged for management of the DCN, which can include both medical and surgical options.
- Standardization of definition, nomenclature, classification, and research protocols is needed for further investigations regarding DCN pathogenesis and treatment outcomes.
- The term diabetic Charcot-Jordan foot better describes the disease and avoids misnomers when managing foot and ankle neuroarthropathy joints in patients with diabetic neuropathy since first described by Jordan in 1936.

In every medical and surgical specialty there exist pathologic conditions that continue to confound even the most experienced individuals and, for foot and ankle surgeons, the diabetic Charcot neuroarthropathy (DCN) is an example. With its variety of unique clinical manifestations and still unknown true pathogenesis, DCN represents an elusive entity despite having numerous proposed medical and surgical treatment options becoming available over the years. An in-depth look into the history of DCN, including diagnostic and therapeutic developments over the last 80 years, demonstrates how much knowledge has been gained but also sheds light onto how much is still needed to go on with continued research into this complex disorder.

Although the name of the overall condition is historically attributed to Jean-Martin Charcot, it is William Riely Jordan[1] who is credited for first establishing an association

---

Disclosure: The authors have nothing to disclose. T. Zgonis is the Consulting Editor for the *Clinics in Podiatric Medicine and Surgery*.
Division of Podiatric Medicine and Surgery, Department of Orthopaedics, University of Texas Health Science Center San Antonio, 7703 Floyd Curl Drive MSC 7776, San Antonio, TX 78229, USA
* Corresponding author.
E-mail address: zgonis@uthscsa.edu

Clin Podiatr Med Surg 34 (2017) 1–8
http://dx.doi.org/10.1016/j.cpm.2016.07.001

between diabetes mellitus and painless Charcot joint of the ankle in 1936. In his article, a 56-year-old woman with a history of 14 years of diabetes mellitus, presented with a "useless and instable"[1] ankle joint that was also found in the contralateral ankle and foot. Two years after the original incidence, a "painless Charcot joint of the ankle in addition to chronic osteomyelitis of the foot of an unusual type and without obvious etiology"[1] was observed and considered "tentatively as a diabetic process of a neurologic trophic nature."[1]

In 1868, Jean-Martin Charcot first described progressive arthropathic joint changes in tabes dorsalis (neurosyphilis) patients.[2] In 1883, even though Jean-Martin Charcot described neuropathic arthropathy of the foot in patients with tabes dorsalis, there is literature to suggest that Herbert William Page was the first individual to describe tabetic neuroarthropathy in the foot and ankle.[2,3] **Box 1** outlines the years of groundwork on neuropathic arthropathy that was initially laid by William Musgrave, John Kearsley Mitchell, Silas Weir Mitchell, Jean-Martin Charcot, and Herbert William Page before William Riely Jordan's discovery in a patient with diabetes mellitus.[4,5]

Since 1936, a plethora of publications have associated the Charcot joint with diabetic neuropathy and specifically in the foot and ankle.[6] In 1937, Dreyfus and Zarachovitch[7] published the second case, followed by Bailey and Root[8,9] in 1942 and 1947, Jordan[10] in 1943, Foster and Bassett[11] in 1947, Morris[12] in 1947, Muri[13] in 1949, Wilson and colleagues[14] in 1949, and many others after 1950. In addition, after Jordan's discovery of the diabetic Charcot joint in the foot and ankle in 1936, multiple diabetic neuroarthropathy anatomic locations have been described, including the knee and spine.[6,15,16]

DESCRIPTION

Quickly following the time of Jordan's observation, additional cases of diabetic Charcot foot and ankle populated the literature.[6–14] However, efforts to classify the stages of Charcot neuroarthropathy (CN) of the foot and ankle were not published until

Box 1
Historical timeline for landmarks in the study of neuroarthropathy

William Musgrave, 1703

- First described neuropathic joint as arthralgia caused by venereal disease

John Kearsley Mitchell, 1827

- Examined spinal origin of rheumatism suggesting relationship between spinal cord lesion and foot and/or ankle arthropathy

Silas Weir Mitchell, 1864

- Described alterations in nutrition of joints related to nerve injuries

Jean-Martin Charcot, 1868

- Described general arthropathies associated with syphilis (tabes dorsalis)

Herbert William Page, 1883

- Earliest description of a rocker-bottom foot deformity associated with a tabetic (syphilitic) arthropathy

William Riely Jordan, 1936

- First established link between foot and/or ankle neuroarthropathy and diabetes mellitus

1966. Sidney N. Eichenholtz[17] defined 3 stages using clinical, radiographic, and histopathologic data of 68 consecutive patients. In 1990, Shibata and colleagues[18] modified the Eichenholtz classification system recognizing a stage 0 CN with clinical signs that precede the radiographic findings typically associated with stage 1 CN. The finding of this prodromal stage has significantly affected therapeutic options in efforts to prevent the development of skeletal destruction and deformity found in subsequent stages. Several other systems have been reported since then, many based on anatomic schemes and imaging findings, yet none have been validated to date.

Current data suggest that CN affects approximately 1% of people with diabetes; however, the prevalence for DCN is likely higher than originally thought due to many cases going undiagnosed or misdiagnosed. Nonetheless, even the estimate of 1% is alarming considering that, according to the International Diabetes Foundation, there are more than 300 million people living with diabetes worldwide. Epidemiologic data for DCN are difficult to interpret based on the wide range of descriptions in the literature. Currently, there are ongoing efforts to standardize the definition, nomenclature, description, and classification of DCN alone because its manifestations and management options are often interpreted and treated differently by physicians and surgeons, making comparisons difficult among studies.

In 1868, Jean-Martin Charcot supported the French Theory for the pathogenesis of CN that proposed that a spinal cord lesion produced the trophic changes seen in the joints.[19] The German Theory, supported by Volkman and Virchow, proposed that CN was due to microtrauma in the insensate limb.[20] The neurovascular theory postulates that autonomic neuropathy predisposes to CN foot via increased blood flow and increased bone resorption. Although the precise pathogenesis is still unknown, current evidence supports that for DCN of the foot and/or ankle to occur, the patient should have diabetic peripheral neuropathy to enhance a local inflammatory response triggered by minor trauma, infection, surgery, or ulceration.[21]

DIAGNOSIS

Descriptions for the physical presentation of early stages in DCN have not changed over the years, including a unilateral warm, edematous, sometimes painful foot and/or ankle. Chronic DCN can manifest with stable or unstable deformities, subluxations, or dislocations at multiple joints of the foot and/or ankle. Soft tissue and/or osseous infection in the presence of ulceration can accompany DCN, further challenging accurate diagnosis and treatment. Laboratory results in DCN are usually equivocal. Although most of the early work in the diagnosis of the DCN foot was based on plain film radiographs, technological advances have led to other more sensitive and specific imaging options. MRI has become the modality of choice in detecting early DCN with significant bone marrow edema changes. Computed tomography (CT) with 3-dimensional visualization has been useful for surgical preoperative planning. Advanced imaging through nuclear medicine and, more recently, with PET combined with CT has shown promising results, especially with regard to DCN complicated by osteomyelitis.[22]

THERAPEUTIC CONSIDERATIONS

Treatment of acute stages of DCN is immediate off-loading. In the nineteenth century, this came in the form of bedrest, compression bandaging, and nonweightbearing plaster casts. Today casting of the lower extremity still remains most effective, with weightbearing and nonweightbearing casts showing similar results.[23] The development of more advanced bracing, such as ankle-foot-orthosis (AFO), patellar-tendon-bearing (PTB) brace, Charcot restraint orthotic walker (CROW), and the removable cast walker provide additional options. However, their usefulness is mostly found in later stages of DCN or even following surgical reconstruction.[24] More recently, surgical intervention during the acute stages of DCN have been described to stabilize the foot and/or ankle with either internal or external fixation to prevent further deformity or destruction, yet only studies with low levels of evidence are available with regard to these approaches.[23]

In attempts to reduce bone turnover in acute DCN, several studies have used bisphosphonates for adjunctive treatment of these patients; however, the results have been inconclusive.[25] Electrical bone stimulation, first developed in the 1950s, has been demonstrated as a useful adjunct in the treatment of acute DCN, as well as in conjunction with surgical reconstruction for chronic DCN, yet the magnitude of benefit is still unknown.[26,27] Newer drug research is focused on therapies that may be able to target inflammatory mediators in the early stages of the condition. Surgical reconstruction for chronic DCN has become more popular in recent decades with several choices, including but not limited to internal fixation (screws, plates, intramedullary nailing, or beaming), external fixation (circular, hybrid, or computer-based constructs), and a combination of internal and external fixation. In cases of concomitant osteomyelitis and wounds, staged reconstruction is often performed with multiple debridements, negative pressure wound therapy, temporary stabilization, use of systemic and local antibiotics, and plastic surgical techniques.[28–30] Unfortunately, most of the existing studies regarding surgical options lack consistency in many areas, including definition and location of DCN, number of subjects, clinical indications for surgical reconstruction, fixation techniques, and long-term outcomes. **Fig. 1** provides some of the available options used for treatment of various clinical manifestations of DCN in the foot and/or ankle.

PROGNOSIS

Despite the increase in published literature over the last 2 decades regarding the DCN, reliable long-term prognostic studies are few and far between. In 2004, Gazis and colleagues[31] demonstrated no difference in mortality rates between patients with DCN and those with uncomplicated neuropathic ulceration. In 2009, Sohn and colleagues[32] found that DCN was significantly associated with higher mortality risk than diabetes alone and with lower risk than foot ulceration. In 2010, Sohn and colleagues[33] concluded that DCN by itself does not have a high lower extremity amputation risk but ulceration with DCN multiplicatively increases amputation risk. These aforementioned studies only included subjects treated by nonsurgical means. In 2015, Ramanujam and colleagues[34] analyzed the morbidity (lower extremity amputation, below-knee amputation) and mortality with surgical reconstruction of the DCN foot and/or ankle with circular external fixation, and found that lower extremity amputation was associated with gender, coronary artery disease, previous vascular intervention, and additional surgery following removal of circular external fixation; whereas mortality was associated with higher body-mass index, coronary artery disease, and additional surgery after removal of circular external fixation. Furthermore, mortality rate for DCN with osteomyelitis was higher than DCN without osteomyelitis. Overall, the morbidity and mortality rate found in this study was low, demonstrating the importance of careful patient selection for DCN surgical reconstruction.

ACCURATE NOMENCLATURE

Jean-Martin Charcot has been named as the father of neurology, providing knowledge and training to notable physicians such as Sigmund Freud and Charles Babinski.[2]

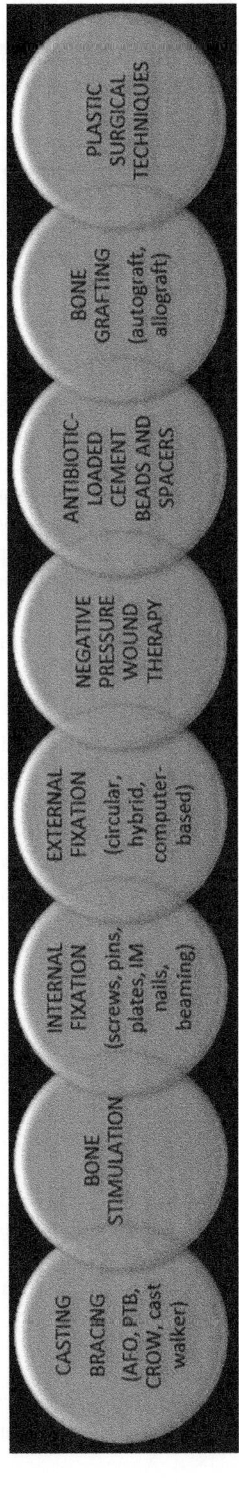

Fig. 1. Options for management of the diabetic Charcot-Jordan foot. IM, intramedullary.

Under his name and legacy, multiple Charcot eponyms have been described and credited to his work.[35] He was known for treating patients with hysteria by using the technique of hypnosis and was given the nicknames of Napoleon of the neurosis[35] and Caesar of the Salpêtrière,[35] the hospital where he worked in Paris, France.

Some of the Charcot eponyms include but are not limited to Charcot's Joint, Charcot's Disease, Charcot-Marie-Tooth Disease, Charcot biliary triad, Charcot cerebral triad, Charcot-Bouchard aneurysm, and Erb-Charcot paralysis.[35] For the diabetic patient with neuroarthropathy of the foot and/or ankle, a universal and accurate description of the pathologic condition will lead to a better consensus for future research and treatment in this specific population. The new term of diabetic Charcot-Jordan foot will be used to describe the pathologic conditions in any foot and/or ankle joints, signifying its findings in only patients with diabetic neuropathy. This will further avoid any confusion with CN patients based on chronic conditions such as leprosy, syphilis, alcoholism, congenital insensitivity to pain, peripheral nerve lesions, idiopathic neuropathy, and others. The literature since Jean-Martin Charcot's findings in 1868 has been fulfilled with numerous nomenclatures, misdiagnoses, tests, and nonconsensus treatments based on the patient's pathologic complications and condition. Diabetic patients with diabetic Charcot-Jordan foot disease represent a unique subspecialty group due to the severity of the condition associated with the presence of medical comorbidities such as vasculopathy, peripheral neuropathy, nephropathy, retinopathy, cardiac disease, and osteoporosis. This subspecialty group also presents with ulcerations, septic arthritis, and concomitant osteomyelitis, making the diagnosis and treatment a challenge to the medical and surgical services.

SUMMARY

The investigations surrounding DCN highlight that a multidisciplinary approach is critical to fully understanding and successfully treating this complex disorder. Although knowledge of DCN has been significantly enhanced through numerous developments over the past 80 years, there are still many questions to be answered, including how to prevent the condition. Future research would benefit from an international consensus on accurate and universal DCN nomenclature, definition, classification, and treatment indications, in addition to standardized techniques and outcome measures.

REFERENCES

1. Jordan WR. Neuritic manifestations in diabetes mellitus. Arch Intern Med 1936; 56:307–66.
2. Kumar DR, Aslinia F, Yale SH, et al. Jean-Martin Charcot: the father of neurology. Clin Med Res 2011;9:46–9.
3. Sanders LJ, Edmonds ME, Jeffcoate WJ. Who was the first to diagnose and report neuropathic arthropathy of the foot and ankle: Jean-martin Charcot or Herbert William Page? Diabetologia 2013;56:873–7.
4. Sanders LJ. The Charcot foot: historical perspective 1827-2003. Diabetes Metab Res Rev 2004;20:S4–8.
5. Kelly M. William Musgrave's De Arthritide Symptomatica (1703): his description of neuropathic arthritis. Bull Hist Med 1963;37:372–6.
6. Robillard R, Gagnon PA, Alarie R. Diabetic neuroarthropathy: report of four cases. Can Med Assoc J 1964;91:795–804.
7. Dreyfus G, Zarachovitch M. Gros orteil d'apparance syringomyelique avec fractures spontanees multiples du metatarse. Bull Med Soc Med Hop Paris 1937;53:328.

8. Bailey CC, Root HF. Neuropathic joint lesions in diabetes mellitus. J Clin Invest 1942;21:649.
9. Bailey CC, Root HF. Neuropathic foot lesions in diabetes mellitus. N Engl J Med 1947;236:397–401.
10. Jordan WR. Effect of diabetes on the nervous system. South Med J 1943;36:45–9.
11. Foster DB, Bassett RC. Neurogenic arthropathy (Charcot joint) associated with diabetic neuropathy; a report of two cases. Arch Neurol Psychiatry 1947;57: 173–85.
12. Morris MH. Charcot's joint in diabetes mellitus. N Y State J Med 1947;47:1395.
13. Muri J. Diabetic arthropathy and intercapillary glomerulonecrosis. Report of a case. Acta Med Scand 1949;135:391–8.
14. Wilson IH, McIntyre CH, Albertson HK. Charcot's joint, with unusual features, in a diabetic patient. Calif Med 1949;70:420–2.
15. De Takats G. Peripheral neurovascular lesions in diabetics. Proc Amer Diabetes Assoc 1945;5:181.
16. Zucker G, Marder MJ. Charcot spine due to diabetic neuropathy. Am J Med 1952; 12:118–24.
17. Eichenholtz SN. Charcot joints. Springfield (IL): Charles C. Thomas; 1966.
18. Shibata T, Tada K, Hashizume C. The results of arthrodesis of the ankle for leprotic neuroarthropathy. J Bone Joint Surg Am 1990;72:749–56.
19. Charcot JM. Sur quelques arthropathies quiparaissent depender d'une lesion du cerneau dela moelle epiniere. Arch Des Physiol Normet Path 1868;1:161 [in French].
20. Delano PJ. The pathogenesis of Charcot's joint. Am J Roentgenol 1946;56: 189–200.
21. Kaynak G, Birsel O, Güven MF, et al. An overview of the Charcot foot pathophysiology. Diabet Foot Ankle 2013;2:4.
22. Pickwell KM, van Kroonenburgh MJ, Weijers RE, et al. F-18 FDG PET/CT scanning in Charcot disease: a brief report. Clin Nucl Med 2011;36:8–10.
23. Schade VL, Andersen CA. A literature-based guide to the conservative and surgical management of the acute Charcot foot and ankle. Diabet Foot Ankle 2015;19:6.
24. Koller A, Meissner SA, Podella M, et al. Orthotic management of Charcot feet after external fixation surgery. Clin Podiatr Med Surg 2007;24:583–99.
25. Richard JL, Almasri M, Schuldiner S. Treatment of acute Charcot foot with bisphosphonates: a systematic review of the literature. Diabetologia 2012;55: 1258–64.
26. Hanft JR, Goggin JP, Landsman A, et al. The role of combined magnetic field bone growth stimulation as an adjunct in the treatment of neuroarthropathy/Charcot joint: an expanded pilot study. J Foot Ankle Surg 1998;37:510–5.
27. Hockenbury RT, Gruttadauria M, McKinney I. Use of implantable bone growth stimulation in Charcot ankle arthrodesis. Foot Ankle Int 2007;28:971–6.
28. Dalla Paola L, Brocco E, Ceccacci T, et al. Limb salvage in Charcot foot and ankle osteomyelitis: combined use single stage/double stage of arthrodesis and external fixation. Foot Ankle Int 2009;30:1065–70.
29. Ramanujam CL, Stapleton JJ, Zgonis T. Negative-pressure wound therapy in the management of diabetic Charcot foot and ankle wounds. Diabet Foot Ankle 2013;23:4.
30. Ramanujam CL, Stapleton JJ, Zgonis T. Diabetic charcot neuroarthropathy of the foot and ankle with osteomyelitis. Clin Podiatr Med Surg 2014;31:487–92.

31. Gazis A, Pound N, Macfarlane R, et al. Mortality in patients with diabetic neuropathic osteoarthropathy (Charcot foot). Diabet Med 2004;21:1243–6.
32. Sohn MW, Lee TA, Stuck RM, et al. Mortality risk of Charcot arthropathy compared with that of diabetic foot ulcer and diabetes alone. Diabetes Care 2009;32:816–21.
33. Sohn MW, Stuck RM, Pinzur M, et al. Lower-extremity amputation risk after charcot arthropathy and diabetic foot ulcer. Diabetes Care 2010;33:98–100.
34. Ramanujam CL, Han D, Zgonis T. Lower extremity amputation and mortality rates in the reconstructed diabetic charcot foot and ankle with external fixation: data analysis of 116 patients. Foot Ankle Spec 2015;9(2):113–26.
35. Kundu AK. Charcot in medical eponyms. J Assoc Physicians India 2004;52:716–8.

Medical Imaging in Differentiating the Diabetic Charcot Foot from Osteomyelitis

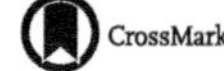

Daniel J. Short, DPM, Thomas Zgonis, DPM*

KEYWORDS

• Diabetic Charcot foot • Charcot neuroarthropathy • Osteomyelitis • Medical imaging • MRI • Computed tomography • Bone scan • Diabetic neuropathy

KEY POINTS

- Plain radiographs can provide the reconstructive surgeon valuable information about the severity of the diabetic Charcot neuroarthropathy (DCN) deformity, anatomic location, osteomyelitis, and soft tissue emphysema.
- Magnetic resonance imaging (MRI) is a great tool for confirming and detecting the early stages of acute DCN with multiple occult fractures and bone marrow edema locations.
- Computed tomography provides a preoperative tool for assessing the multiplane deformity and planning for correction of the underlying deformity.
- Advanced bone scintigraphy may be used to further differentiate between DCN and concomitant osteomyelitis with intraoperative bone biopsy and histopathologic analysis being the test of choice to confirm a diagnosis.

Neurotrophic osteoarthropathy was originally described by a French neurologist Jean-Martin Charcot in 1868 with an association to syphilis.[1] William Riely Jordan was the first to associate the clinical entity with diabetes mellitus in 1936.[2] Although almost 150 years have passed since the initial description of the disease, diabetic Charcot neuroarthropathy (DCN) continues to challenge clinicians from all disciplines. Keys to management include early detection, stabilization/offloading of the extremity, and prevention of the destruction of foot architecture. If allowed to continue through its natural clinical course, progressive destruction of normal joint alignment produces

---

Disclosure: The authors have nothing to disclose. T. Zgonis is the Consulting Editor for the Clinics in Podiatric Medicine and Surgery.
Reconstructive Foot and Ankle Surgery, Division of Podiatric Medicine and Surgery, Department of Orthopaedics, University of Texas Health Science Center San Antonio, 7703 Floyd Curl Drive, MSC 7776, San Antonio, TX 78229, USA
* Corresponding author.
E-mail address: zgonis@uthscsa.edu

Clin Podiatr Med Surg 34 (2017) 9–14
http://dx.doi.org/10.1016/j.cpm.2016.07.002 podiatric.theclinics.com
0891-8422/17/

osseous prominences that, coupled with peripheral neuropathy, can lead to ulceration, infection, and amputation. The goal of DCN management is to provide a stable lower extremity free of ulceration and/or infection while allowing the patient to maintain a level of independence with ambulatory status.

When DCN presents with an ulceration and/or concomitant osteomyelitis, initial medical imaging of plain radiographs to magnetic resonance imaging (MRI) and computed tomography (CT) can become quite challenging to differentiate between DCN and concomitant infection. Advanced nuclear imaging (NI) may provide a great tool when dealing with the complex DCN with concomitant osteomyelitis. This article reviews a variety of medical imaging techniques currently available to the clinician with a focus on early detection, differentiation between DCN and osteomyelitis, and monitoring of the DCN foot.

PLAIN RADIOGRAPHS AND THE DIABETIC CHARCOT FOOT

Plain radiographs are part of the initial first line testing in the workup when concern for DCN foot and ankle deformities. Plain radiographs, including foot, ankle, calcaneal, and lower extremity views, are preferred to be taken in a weight-bearing status when feasible for assessing the multilevel deformities associated with the DCN. Plain radiographs can provide initial valuable information including and not limited to anatomic location, severity of joint fragmentation and fracture/dislocation, presence of osteomyelitis and/or soft tissue emphysema, or presence of foreign bodies. Few studies have been attempted to establish radiographic parameters to predict development of ulceration in midfoot DCN. Although a definitive threshold has not been established, the work does show that sagittal plane deformities have a higher incidence of ulceration when compared with transverse plane deformity.[3,4]

In 1976, Classen and colleagues[5] showed the red, hot, swollen Charcot foot precedes any changes on imaging studies. However, many entities can cause the same clinical picture, which can often lead to a misdiagnosis and delay in treatment. The most common differential diagnoses associated with the acute DCN include and are not limited to cellulitis, deep vein thrombosis, osteomyelitis, gout, sprain, and stress fractures. Plain radiographs have been shown to have very poor sensitivity and specificity (<50%) in detecting early DCN changes, necessitating advanced medical imaging.[6] Additionally, once signs of fracture and dislocation are visible on plain radiographs, the process has advanced to later stages of DCN and the focus of clinical care shifts from prevention of fracture and dislocation to management of deformity. Severe initial deformity or progressive collapse on serial plain radiographs, combined with clinical joint instability, presence of osseous prominence with partial thickness overlying tissue, or preulcerative lesions, may indicate early surgical intervention to prevent ulceration rather than using pure radiographic assessments (**Fig. 1**A–F).

MRI AND COMPUTED TOMOGRAPHY SCANS FOR THE DIABETIC CHARCOT FOOT

MRI has been shown to be the most reliable method for evaluating an early DCN without fracture/dislocation and when osseous fragmentation is not visible with plain radiographs. MRI characteristic findings for DCN are subchondral bone marrow edema with minimal amounts of joint fluid.[7] However, an early MRI detection for DCN requires a musculoskeletal radiologist with experience in neuroathropathy of the foot and ankle. If early detection of DCN can be achieved, immediate offloading and/or immobilization has been shown to prevent the progression of the DCN deformity.[8,9]

Any bone marrow edema on an MRI, regardless of its causative factor, in an insensate foot with swelling has the ability to progress frank cortical fracture if allowed to

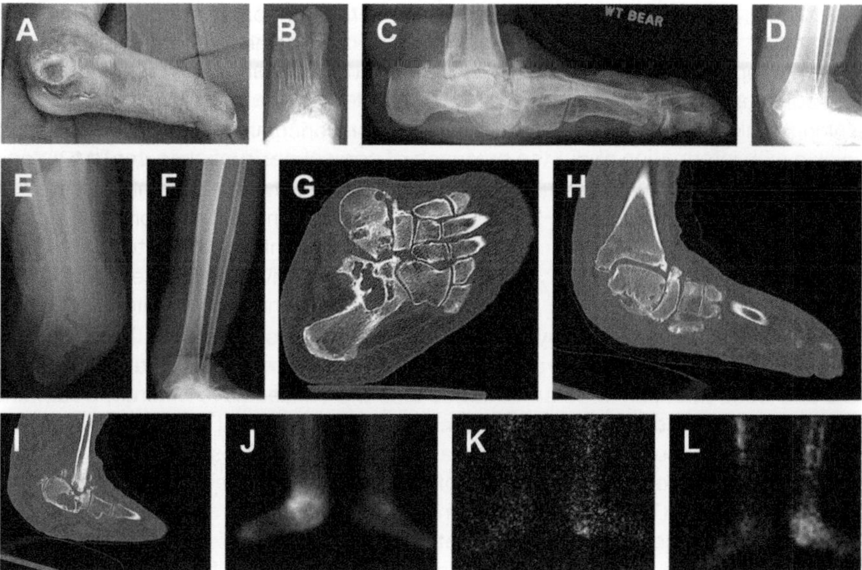

Fig. 1. Preoperative clinical (*A*) and radiographic foot (*B, C*), ankle (*D*), calcaneal (*E*), and leg (*F*) views showing a severe diabetic Charcot neuroathropathy with chromic open wound concerned for concomitant osteomyelitis. The patient underwent a computed tomography (CT) scan to further evaluate the deformity for preoperative planning and also assess for any soft tissue emphysema and cortical destruction that might be indicative of osteomyelitis (*G–I*). The CT scan results were negative for osteomyelitis showing the ulceration with severe diabetic Charcot neuroarthropathy deformity at multiple foot and ankle locations. Further nuclear imaging including a technetium-99m (Tc-99m) followed by a leukocyte imaging with indium-111 and bone marrow sulfur colloid were also performed to assess for concomitant osteomyelitis. Note the increased uptake of the blood pool phase Tc-99m study (*J*), followed by an increased uptake indium-111 (*K*) and increased uptake sulfur colloid scans (*L*). The 3-phase Tc-99m was found to have an increase uptake in various anatomic locations of the foot and ankle, whereas both the indium-111 and bone marrow sulfur colloid scans had an increased uptake in the talus and calcaneus indicating no evidence of osteomyelitis. These findings were also confirmed with an intraoperative bone biopsy and histopathological analysis not consistent with acute osteomyelitis even though intraoperative soft tissue and bone cultures were positive for aerobic and anaerobic bacteria.

remain exposed to repeated stress.[10–13] Osseous inflammation, either sterile or septic, produces skeletal fragility, thereby increasing the susceptibility to injury from normal weight bearing.[9] In the initial detection of bone marrow edema associated with DCN, offloading of the involved extremity can prevent the development of DCN as a result of the increased local inflammation and compromised osseous integrity.

MRI continues to have the ability to evaluate changes of DCN with bone marrow edema and occult fracture as well as evaluate for any concomitant soft tissue injury. In the absence of an ulceration and/or osteomyelitis, MRI can be a great tool for the early detection of DCN if it cannot be diagnosed with plain radiographs. In addition, it can also be used for the assessment of any soft tissue injury, including and not limited to ligamentous and tendinous structures that can provide instability to the neuropathic foot. However, MRI can be quite challenging when dealing with the ulcerated and/or infected DCN because findings might be similar when DCN and osteomyelitis coexist.

CT imaging for the DCN has a role in evaluating the extent and involvement of fractures and/or dislocations and serve as a great tool for preoperative planning of the deformity correction. Advancement of 3-dimensional reconstruction technology, digital imaging, and digital templates allow for accurate and reliable preoperative surgical planning, which adds to the effectiveness of CT scans. CT scans can also provide the clinician with information about the presence of cortical destruction to confirm osteomyelitis or soft tissue emphysema when an open wound and/or osteomyelitis is also involved with the DCN (**Fig. 1**G–I).

NUCLEAR IMAGING FOR THE DIABETIC CHARCOT FOOT

When the DCN is complicated by an open wound and/or osteomyelitis, the diagnostic challenge to the clinician is increased significantly. Accurate differentiation between DCN and bone infection is paramount because the entities have different treatment protocols. Further confounding the diagnostic dilemma is that these 2 entities can often be found simultaneously in the same foot, and that osteomyelitis has also been shown to trigger the development of neurotrophic changes.[14–17]

Technetium-99m (Tc-99m) NI has a limited role in both the early stages of acute DCN where its use cannot differentiate between other pathologies within the differential diagnosis, and in the attempt to differentiate between DCN from osteomyelitis by itself. However, other advanced NI techniques are able to provide increased specificity making them more valuable to the clinician.

One such NI technique includes labeled white blood cell bone scans. This process involves taking a sample of the patient's blood, separating the white blood cells and processing them so they are tagged with a radiotracer, either indium-111 or Tc-99m. The tagged white blood cells are then injected back into the patient and before the medical imaging begin in multiple stages. Accumulation of the tagged radiotracer in the area of clinical interest is indicative of infection, but this finding may be challenging in the presence of DCN with or without osteomyelitis. Leukocyte imaging with indium-111 or Tc-99m has varying reported sensitivities and specificities for detection of osteomyelitis ranging from 50% to 100% and 29% to 100%, respectively.[18]

In some cases, increased labeled white blood cell accumulation may also be observed in fracture sites of patients with DCN. The exact reason is unclear and is likely multifactorial. This phenomenon was initially attributed to the localized inflammation and fractures associated with DCN but the inflammatory response involved with a fracture is polymorphonuclear only in its early phases.[19] In addition, significant challenge are encountered when the leukocyte NI is positive in the presence of DCN and concomitant osteomyelitis. In these unique cases, combined imaging techniques with Tc-99m sulfur colloid may increase the specificity of differentiating between DCN and osteomyelitis. In osteomyelitis, white blood cell uptake is stimulated, whereas sulfur colloid uptake is suppressed. The white blood cell–labeled bone marrow study is positive for osteomyelitis when there is activity on the white blood cell image without corresponding activity on the bone marrow image. Any other pattern of the white blood cell–labeled bone marrow study is negative for infection. Combining white blood cell labeled and sulfur colloid bone scans have reported promising results (**Fig. 1**J–L).[20]

The use of fluorodeoxyglucose (FDG) PET is an NI technique that uses FDG, a marker of increased intracellular glucose metabolism.[21] FDG uptake is increased in both infection and DCN.[21] Combined with high resolution imaging, FDG-PET has shown promising results in the diagnosis of osteomyelitis of the diabetic foot and has become more widely used owing to the ability of quantifying results. One study, comparing FDG-PET and MRI with histopathologic results, showed the average standard uptake value was 1.3 ± 0.4 compared with 4.38 ± 1.39 in osteomyelitis.[22] When Charcot and osteomyelitis were both present, the standardized uptake value was 6.5. This study showed overall sensitivity and accuracy for diagnosing Charcot foot was 100% and 93.8%, whereas MRI was 76.9% and 75%, respectively.[22]

One of the most important aspects of FDG-PET is its high negative predictive value throughout all stages that can rule out DCN and osteomyelitis. Some disadvantages of FDG-PET imaging include the limited availability of the technology compared with other modalities, such as plain radiographs, MRI, CT, and conventional NI as well as the high cost of completing the scans.

DISCUSSION

Although multiple medical imaging studies are available in the early or late DCN stages, differentiating between DCN and osteomyelitis or identifying the presence of DCN with concomitant infection becomes a great challenge for the nuclear medicine radiologists and clinicians. Early and accurate medical imaging diagnosis along with a thorough history and physical examination are paramount to the patient's successful treatment. MRI is greatly beneficial in the early detection of DCN and when there is high clinical index of suspicion not identifiable in plain radiographs. MRI can also be used in monitoring the resolution of bone marrow edema, but how this correlates to the risk of fracture or recurrence of the disease is unclear. CT imaging may be a great preoperative tool for assessing the multiplane DCN deformity before surgical reconstruction and realignment. Advanced bone scintigraphy has shown to have promising results in differentiating between DCN and/or osteomyelitis whereas intraoperative bone biopsy, bone cultures, and histopathologic analysis may still be the most reliable tests for identifying the underlying pathology.

SUMMARY

Although Charcot foot pathology was originally described almost 150 years ago, there is surprisingly minimal consensus on the etiology, pathophysiology, and current treatments for the DCN. Although DCN is still considered a rare disease process, the potential implications of the development and progression of deformity has significant implications for the patient and the health care system at large. Necessary future research includes large cohort direct comparison studies of available medical imaging modalities.

REFERENCES

1. Charcot J. Sur quelques arthropathies qui paraissent dependre d'une lesion du cerveau ou de la moelle epiniere. Arch Physiol Norm Pathol 1868;1:161–78.
2. Jordan WR. Neuritic manifestations in diabetes mellitus. Arch Intern Med 1936; 57:307–66.
3. Wukich DK, Raspovic KM, Hobizal KB, et al. Radiographic analysis of diabetic midfoot Charcot neuroarthropathy with and without midfoot ulceration. Foot Ankle Int 2014;35:1108–15.
4. Bevan WP, Tomlinson MP. Radiographic measures as a predictor of ulcer formation in diabetic Charcot midfoot. Foot Ankle Int 2008;29:568–73.
5. Classen JN, Rolley RT, Carneiro R, et al. Management of foot conditions of the diabetic patient. Am Surg 1976;42:81–8.

6. Sanverdi SE, Ergen BF, Oznur A. Current challenges in imaging of the diabetic foot. Diabet Foot Ankle 2012;3. http://dx.doi.org/10.3402/dfa.v3i0.18754.
7. Mautone M, Naidoo P. What the radiologist needs to know about Charcot foot. J Med Imaging Radiat Oncol 2015;59:395–402.
8. Chantelau EA, Grützner G. Is the Eichenholtz classification still valid for the diabetic Charcot foot? Swiss Med Wkly 2014;144:w13948.
9. Chantelau EA, Richter A. The acute diabetic Charcot foot managed on the basis of magnetic resonance imaging–a review of 71 cases. Swiss Med Wkly 2013;143: w13831.
10. Weishaupt D, Schweitzer ME, Alam F, et al. Imaging of inflammatory joint diseases of the foot and ankle. Skeletal Radiol 1999;28:663–9.
11. Weishaupt D, Schweitzer ME. MR imaging of the foot and ankle: patterns of bone marrow signal abnormalities. Eur Radiol 2002;12:416–26.
12. Rios AM, Rosenberg ZS, Bencardino JT, et al. Bone marrow edema patterns in the ankle and hindfoot: distinguishing MRI features. Am J Roentgenol 2011; 197:W720–9.
13. Teh J, Suppiah R, Sharp R, et al. Imaging in the assessment and management of overuse injuries in the foot and ankle. Semin Musculoskelet Radiol 2011;15: 101–14.
14. Aragón-Sánchez J, Lázaro-Martínez JL, Hernández-Herrero MJ. Triggering mechanisms of neuroarthropathy following conservative surgery for osteomyelitis. Diabet Med 2010;27:844–7.
15. Aragón-Sánchez J, Lázaro-Martínez JL, Quintana-Marrero Y, et al. Charcot neuroarthropathy triggered and complicated by osteomyelitis. How limb salvage can be achieved. Diabet Med 2013;30:e229–32.
16. Ndip A, Jude EB, Whitehouse R, et al. Charcot neuroarthropathy triggered by osteomyelitis and/or surgery. Diabet Med 2008;25:1469–72.
17. Levitt BA, Stapleton JJ, Zgonis T. Diabetic Lisfranc fracture-dislocations and Charcot neuroarthropathy. Clin Podiatr Med Surg 2013;30:257–63.
18. Wang GL, Zhao K, Liu ZF, et al. A meta-analysis of fluorodeoxyglucose-positron emission tomography versus scintigraphy in the evaluation of suspected osteomyelitis. Nucl Med Commun 2011;32:1134–42.
19. Rosenberg AE. Bones, joints, and soft tissue tumors. In: Kumar V, Abbas AK, Fausto N, editors. Robbins and Cotran pathologic basis of disease. 7th edition. Philadelphia: Elsevier Saunders; 2005. p. 1273–324.
20. Palestro CJ, Mehta HH, Patel M, et al. Marrow versus infection in the Charcot joint: indium-111 leukocyte and technetium-99m sulfur colloid scintigraphy. J Nucl Med 1998;39:346–50.
21. Keidar Z, Militianu D, Melamed E, et al. The diabetic foot: initial experience with 18F-FDG PET/CT. J Nucl Med 2005;46:444–9.
22. Basu S, Chryssikos T, Houseni M, et al. Potential role of FDG PET in the setting of diabetic neuro-osteoarthropathy: can it differentiate uncomplicated Charcot's neuroarthropathy from osteomyelitis and soft-tissue infection? Nucl Med Commun 2007;28:465–72.

Conservative and Pharmacologic Treatments for the Diabetic Charcot Foot

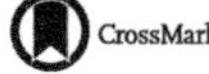

Nina L. Petrova, MD, PhD*, Michael E. Edmonds, MD, FRCP

KEYWORDS

- Charcot neuroarthropathy • Diabetes mellitus • MRI • Casting therapy
- Disease activity

KEY POINTS

- The total contact cast (TCC) is a well-recognized gold standard treatment of the acute Charcot neuroarthropathy or Charcot foot.
- Frequency of use of TCC varies between clinical centers and countries and this treatment modality is still very much underused.
- Novel reliable biomarkers are urgently needed to monitor disease activity and the response to casting therapy.
- Pharmacologic therapies recently used in the management of the Charcot foot do not have proven efficacy and are not recommended for clinical practice.
- A novel therapeutic approach is urgently needed to stave off the pathologic bone destruction of the acute Charcot foot.

INTRODUCTION

Charcot neuroarthropathy or Charcot foot, is a rare but devastating complication of diabetic neuropathy and is associated with enormous morbidity and disability. Diabetic patients with this condition require considerable long-term support and their prognosis is poor. In a summary of 15 published reports, there were 11 deaths in 301 patients in a 2.5-year follow-up and partial or complete foot amputation occurred in 20 of the 301 patients, and 83 of the 301 patients had limitations of mobility,[1] leading to the characterization of patients with Charcot neuroarthropathy as "frail patients with fragile feet."[2] The Charcot foot is associated with reduced quality of life and even increased mortality.[3–5] Moreover, treatment costs of comorbidities associated with a Charcot foot are 17.2% greater compared with treatment costs of patients with

Disclosure Statement: The authors have nothing to disclose.
Diabetic Foot Clinic, King's College Hospital NHS Foundation Trust, Denmark Hill, London SE5 9RS, UK
* Corresponding author.
E-mail address: petrovanl@yahoo.com

Clin Podiatr Med Surg 34 (2017) 15–24
http://dx.doi.org/10.1016/j.cpm.2016.07.003 podiatric.theclinics.com
0891-8422/17/

diabetic peripheral neuropathy alone.[6] Thus, an improved understanding of its pathogenesis, early diagnosis, and timely management are essential to prevent adverse outcomes. This article discusses the presentation and diagnosis of Charcot neuroarthropathy as well as conservative and pharmacologic management of the acute Charcot foot. Finally, it discusses possible future therapies for the management of the Charcot foot.

PRESENTATION AND DIAGNOSIS

The diabetic Charcot foot often presents without warning and can rapidly deteriorate into severe irreversible foot deformity leading to ulceration and sometimes amputation. The incidence of diabetic foot ulceration is 17% per year[7] and the risk of lower extremity amputation is 12 times higher in patients with Charcot foot deformity and ulcer compared with Charcot foot alone.[8]

Charcot foot is a clinical diagnosis and it is necessary to have a high index of suspicion.[9] Attention to detail and a comprehensive medical history are essential. Early signs include redness and swelling of the foot after trivial trauma. These initial signs may be underestimated by the patient because of the coexisting peripheral neuropathy, gait abnormalities, and often impaired vision.[10] At presentation, the foot is warm to the touch and skin foot temperatures measured with an infrared thermometer are greater in the affected foot compared with the contralateral foot.[11] These classical signs may be absent or diminished in patients on posttransplant immunosuppressive therapy.[12]

There are no established biological markers to diagnose the Charcot foot. In patients with clinically suspected Charcot foot, standard weight-bearing foot and ankle radiographs should be always requested to look for evidence of early bone damage and joint malalignment. When patients present in the early stages of the natural history of the disease, initial radiographs may not show the typical radiologic changes of active bone destruction (**Fig. 1**A, B). It is recommended to organize further imaging such as a triphasic technetium disphosphonate bone scan (**Fig. 1**C, D) or a MRI scan (**Fig. 1**E–G) to look actively for bone destruction.[13]

Differential Diagnosis

It is important to differentiate between the red, hot, swollen Charcot foot and the red, hot, swollen cellulitic foot. The serum inflammatory marker C-reactive protein is usually high in infection and only mildly elevated in the acute active stage of the Charcot neuroarthropathy.[14,15] The presence of gout and deep vein thrombosis should also be ruled out by measurement of serum uric acid (which is usually raised in gout) and duplex vein scan.[9]

CONSERVATIVE TREATMENT FOR THE DIABETIC CHARCOT FOOT

Casting Therapy

The gold standard therapy for the management of the active diabetic Charcot foot is offloading with nonremovable total contact cast (TCC). This treatment modality offloads the foot; reduces mechanical forces, edema, and inflammation; redistributes the plantar pressure; and limits bone and joint destruction.[16]

Casting therapy is indicated not only for patients who present with typical radiologic bone and joint destruction, but also in patients who present early with essentially normal pedal radiographs.[17] The latter presentation is now referred to stage 0 or the incipient Charcot foot and is characterized by mild foot swelling and warmth, dilated veins, and some loss of foot contours but no obvious deformity. A favorable outcome has

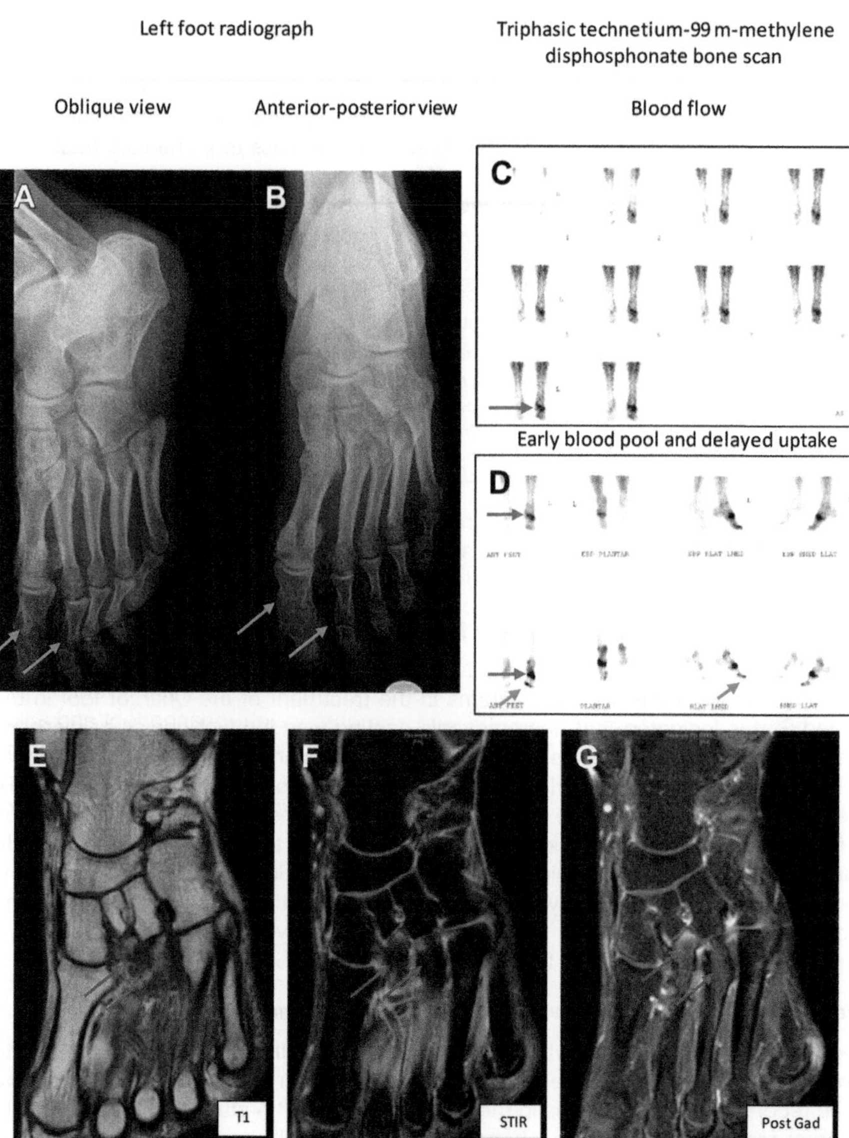

Fig. 1. Foot radiograph (*A, B*), a triphasic technetium-99m-methylene disphosphonate bone scan (*C, D*), and MRI scan of a patient presenting with a hot swollen left foot (*E–G*). Normal alignment of the midfoot with no bone and joint damage of the tarsometatarsal joints noted on the oblique (*A*) and anteroposterior view (*B*) of the left foot radiograph. The bone scan shows an asymmetrical blood flow (left foot > right foot) with acute inflammation in the left foot together with a focal increased uptake in the midfoot (blood flow and early blood pool images; *red arrows* in *C, D*); and increased bone turnover associated with a midfoot lesion at the delayed uptake image (*red arrows* in *D*). In addition, there is radiologic evidence of healed fractures of the first and second toes (*blue arrows* in *A* and *B*), associated with increased bone turnover noted only at the delayed uptake images of the bone scan (*blue arrows* in *D*). Abnormal MRI scan showing subchondral edema with enhancement (*red arrows*) noted at the second and third tarsometatarsal joints on the T1 (*E*), short tau inversion recovery (STIR) sequence with fat suppression, (*F*) and postgadolinium (Post Gad; *G*) images.

been reported in patients in whom casting was initiated early compared with patients with delayed presentation.[18] In patients presenting early with a Charcot foot, casting therapy can arrest the development of foot deformity and progression of the disease.[17]

The success of casting therapy and final clinical outcome (Charcot foot deformity) depend on not only on the time of presentation and access to immediate treatment, but also on the site (forefoot, midfoot, or hindfoot) and the extent of bone and joint involvement. Hindfoot and midfoot involvement requires longer offloading in TCC compared with that of forefoot involvement.[19] Casts should be changed frequently and patients should be encouraged to seek help instantly should any problems occur. Patients should be instructed to look for danger signs (cast breaks, leakage, or staining), to monitor routinely their blood sugars and body temperature, and to present immediately if in doubt about any complications (cast structural problems, unexplained hyperglycemia, and/or fever). A safety network is essential for successful management of this treatment in the diabetic Charcot foot.

DIFFERENCES IN TREATMENT PRACTICES

Although the benefits of casting therapy for the diabetic Charcot foot are well-recognized, this treatment modality is still very much underused and treatment practices vary between clinical centers and countries.

Total Contact Casting as a First Choice Treatment in the Management of the Diabetic Charcot Foot

A recent survey of the practice patterns in the treatment of the Charcot foot in the United States indicated that nonremovable casting was the first choice of management in only 49% of the cases.[20] In the UK, data from an online survey showed that only 34% of patients were offered a nonremovable cast at any one time point for the management of the acute Charcot foot.[21] One of the reasons for this underuse is fear of iatrogenic complications associated with TCC therapy. A recent audit indicated that, with frequent monitoring and patient education, the complication rate is very low.[22] More encouragingly, the majority of complications associated with casting therapy are graded as minor.[23] It is essential that a safety network is in place to reassure the patient and minimize the risk of complications.

Weight-bearing Versus Non–weight-bearing Casting Therapy

There are no firm guidelines whether patients treated with TCC should be allowed to bear weight. Clinical outcomes of patients treated with weight-bearing casts have been reported in 2 small series in the United States.[24,25] A study of 10 patients with Charcot foot in an acute Eichenholtz stage I treated with weight-bearing TCC and biweekly cast changes reported that all subjects were managed successfully and were able to use commercially available depth-inlay shoes and custom accommodative foot orthoses.[24] A further study did not report any deleterious effect from weight-bearing, specifically with regard to skin ulceration or rapid deterioration of the osseous architecture, in 33 of the 34 Charcot feet treated with weight-bearing TCC.[25] In the United States, 41% of orthopedic surgeons have indicated that they manage Charcot feet in weight-bearing casts.[20] Although these series reported data prospectively, a well-controlled clinical trial is needed to fully answer this clinical dilemma.

Duration of Casting Therapy

Practices vary regarding the actual duration of casting therapy. Studies carried out in the UK on average report a longer duration of casting (median of 10 months),[21] compared with studies in the United States (varying between 9 and 16 weeks).[11,24,25] The reason for these differences is unknown, but 1 reason may be the lack of reliable indicators to determine the clinical resolution of the Charcot neuroarthropathy.

So far there have been no suitable markers to monitor the Charcot foot disease activity. The proinflammatory cytokines tumor necrosis factor-α and interleukin-6 have been evaluated prospectively in the natural history of the Charcot foot in patients treated with casting therapy.[26] These cytokines showed a significant reduction from presentation to resolution.[26] In contrast, a more recent study reported a sustained increase of interleukin-6 and tumor necrosis factor-α noted shortly after starting offloading therapy.[27] Moreover, this increase was associated with evidence of accelerated bone healing on foot and ankle radiographs.[27] A further study reported that the acute active stage of Charcot neuroarthropathy is associated with activation of inflammatory and suppression of antiinflammatory cytokines, which reversed at the stage of recovery.[28] Although these studies clearly confirm the role of inflammation in the neuroarthropathy, suitable markers have not been established in everyday clinical practice to measure the activity of Charcot foot disease.

MONITORING OF CASTING THERAPY

Skin Foot Temperature Measurement with an Infrared Thermometry

Foot swelling and skin foot temperatures are traditionally monitored during the course of Charcot foot disease to assess clinical resolution and to help deem that the Charcot foot has progressed from an active into an inactive stage.[29,30] During the treatment phase, a gradual cooling (on average 0.022 ± 0.0005 °C per day) has been noted.[30] It is now established that regular temperature measurements is a useful tool to monitor offloading therapy and a useful aid in making the clinical decision on withdrawal of immobilization.[31]

Doppler Spectrum of the First Dorsal Metatarsal Artery

More recently, blood flow measurements have been used to monitor disease activity and guide treatment. In the acute active stage, the Doppler spectrum of the first dorsal metatarsal artery of the affected Charcot foot showed monophasic forward flow. All patients were treated in a well-padded non–weight-bearing cast until the Doppler spectrum patterns returned to normal after a mean of 13.6 weeks (range, 6–20) of immobilization.[32]

Serial Imaging

Serial imaging (radiographs and MRI scans) is an essential tool in the management of the Charcot foot. Standard weight-bearing foot and ankle radiographs show structural changes and progression of deformity in the natural history of the disease.[33] More recently, serial MRI scans have been used because they show a strong correlation with clinical findings[34] and provide important information on the extent of bone injury in the diabetic Charcot foot.[35] Thus, in the last decade MRI scans have been increasingly used in the monitoring of treatment.[35]

Future Questions Related to Casting Therapy that Remain to Be Answered

- Efficacy of removable versus nonremoval casts.
- Benefits/pitfalls in using weight-bearing versus non–weight-bearing casts.
- Reliable biomarkers to monitor the Charcot foot disease activity.
- Quantitative imaging methods to guide clinicians with regard to resolution of the Charcot neuroarthropathy.

REHABILITATION FROM CASTING THERAPY TO FOOTWEAR

The transition from casting therapy to shoes is a crucial element in the treatment and is equally important to the overall outcome as the casting therapy itself. Patients should be measured for bespoke footwear once the swelling is reduced, the radiographs show evidence of consolidation and the foot is no longer changing shape.

Casting immobilization should be followed by a gradual rehabilitation from cast treatment to suitable bespoke footwear. Patients should be provided with a removable bivalve cast or a cast walker and advised to wear the new footwear initially only for a few steps. Patients should be instructed to look specifically for swelling or pain or discomfort while gradually transitioning from cast to footwear and to seek advice immediately if there is concern that the neuroarthropathy has reactivated. The relapse rate can be as high as 30% and some patients may require additional casting therapy. When the patient comes out of the cast, there will be wasting of the calf muscles and joint stiffness. There is no established rehabilitation program for patients with this condition. An individually tailored approach is advisable and this should be based on patient's overall condition and comorbidities. If there is no increase in warmth, swelling, and redness, then the patient can walk a few more steps each day, and very carefully build up to a reasonable amount of walking. Finally, the patient may progress to bespoke footwear with molded insoles.

Another modality used as a transition device is the Charcot restraint orthotic walker.[36] It is particularly useful when controlling leg edema. Its efficacy is not fully established and its use is variable in clinical practice.[36] Once patients have reached the chronic stable stage of Charcot neuroarthropathy, any foot or ankle deformity needs to be accommodated, supported, or corrected. It is important to prevent secondary ulceration, which usually occurs at sites of bony prominences related to the Charcot foot and/or ankle deformity.[2]

PHARMACOLOGIC TREATMENT

There are no established pharmacologic therapies to manage the Charcot foot condition.[37,38] Experience with antiresorptive therapies (osteoclast inhibitors) and anabolic therapies (which increase the production of bone matrix by osteoblasts) has been limited to clinical trials in small cohorts of patients with Charcot neuroarthropathy, and evidence to support their use in clinical practice is weak.[39]

Therapies that have been used in the management of the Charcot foot in addition to casting therapy include treatment with the antiresorptive agents (bisphosphonates and calcitonin) and an anabolic agent (recombinant parathyroid human hormone). The aim of these therapies is to correct the imbalance between the extensive bone resorption of the acute Charcot foot and the impaired bone formation. Indeed, several studies have demonstrated that in the active stage of the Charcot neuroarthropathy, there is increased osteoclastic activity, which is not coupled with an increase in bone formation.[26,40] Overall, this leads to severe bone destruction and fragmentation, delayed fracture healing, and/or fracture nonunion, which is further aggravated on the background of neuropathy and uncontrolled inflammation.[41]

Antiresorptive Agents

Two groups of therapies have been evaluated in the treatment of the acute Charcot foot including intravenous (pamidronate and zolendronate) and oral (alendronate) bisphosphonate,[42–44] and intranasal calcitonin[45] (**Table 1**). Although these systemic antiresorptive therapies clearly demonstrated a significant reduction in bone turnover, they had no efficacy with regard to clinical resolution. None of these therapies showed

Table 1
Antiresorptive therapies in Charcot neuroarthropathy

	Bisphosphonates			Calcitonin
Active substance [Author, Year]	Pamidronate [Jude et al,[42] 2001]	Zolendronate [Pakarinen et al,[43] 2011]	Alendronate [Pitocco et al,[44] 2005]	Calcitonin [Bem et al,[45] 2006]
Study design	Multicenter double-blind randomized controlled trial	Single-center double-blind randomized controlled trial	Single-center randomized controlled trial	Single-center randomized controlled trial
Participants (n)	39	39	20	32
Active/control (n)	21/18	18/17	11/9	16/16
Type 1/type 2 (n)	13/26	17/22	Not reported	21/11
Sex (male/female), n	26/13	26/6	Not reported	11/21
Intervention (active/control)	90 mg Pamidronate (IV)/ placebo	4 mg Zolendronic acid (IV)/ placebo (IV)	70 mg alendronate (oral once a week)/nil	Salmon calcitonin 200 IU (nasal spray) + calcium supplementation (oral)/ calcium supplementation (oral)
Reduction in skin foot temperatures	Nonsignificant	Not reported	Nonsignificant	Nonsignificant
Reduction in bone turnover	Significant	Not reported	Significant	Significant
Improvement in symptoms	Significant	Not reported	Significant	Not reported
Median time of total immobilization	Not reported	Significant 27 wk (active)/20 wk (placebo)	Not reported	Not reported

an effect on temperature reduction between active treatment group and control.[37] Moreover, treatment with zolendronate resulted in longer cast immobilization compared with placebo.[43] Therefore, at present these therapies have not been established as suitable agents in the management of the Charcot foot and are currently not recommended in clinical practice.[39]

Anabolic Therapies

There is limited experience in using human parathyroid hormone in patients with Charcot neuroarthropathy. Recently, a double-blind randomized control study in patients with acute Charcot foot to evaluate the possible benefit of 1 to 84 recombinant human parathyroid hormone on fracture healing has been completed,[30] although results from this clinical trial are still pending.

SUMMARY OF PHARMACOLOGIC THERAPIES AND FUTURE PERSPECTIVES

It is possible that the window of opportunity to administer these therapies is limited. Alternatively, it is possible that the lack of efficacy of these systemic therapies to modulate osteoblastic and osteoclastic activity may be due to their low bioavailability in the affected Charcot bones. This suggests that a higher dose may be required to achieve therapeutic concentration (which may increase their side effects and toxicity).

A novel way to go forward may be a local drug delivery system to the affected bone, because it would require less medication and would in turn reduce both toxicity and side effects.[46] Future studies are needed to explore the best possible agents for targeted therapy and tailored drug delivery systems in the affected Charcot bones.

SUMMARY

An improved understanding of the early presentation and natural history of the acute Charcot foot as well as a multidisciplinary approach to diagnosis and management are the keys in the current standards of Charcot foot management. A novel therapeutic approach is needed for improved outcome of this disabling foot complication of diabetic neuropathy.

REFERENCES

1. Sinacore DR, Withrington NC. Recognition and management of acute neuropathic (Charcot) arthropathies of the foot and ankle. J Orthop Sports Phys Ther 1999;29:736–46.
2. Fabrin J, Larsen K, Holstein PE. Long-term follow-up in diabetic Charcot feet with spontaneous onset. Diabetes Care 2000;23:796–800.
3. Dhawan V, Spratt KF, Pinzur MS, et al. Reliability of AOFAS diabetic foot questionnaire in Charcot arthropathy: stability, internal consistency, and measurable difference. Foot Ankle Int 2005;26:717–31.
4. Gazis A, Pound N, Macfarlane R, et al. Mortality in patients with diabetic neuropathic osteoarthropathy (Charcot foot). Diabet Med 2004;21:1243–6.
5. van Baal J, Hubbard R, Game F, et al. Mortality associated with acute Charcot foot and neuropathic foot ulceration. Diabetes Care 2010;33:1086–9.
6. Labovitz JM, Shofler DW, Ragothaman KK. The impact of comorbidities on inpatient Charcot neuroarthropathy cost and utilization. J Diabet Complications 2015;30(4):710–5.

7. Larsen K, Fabrin J, Holstein PE. Incidence and management of ulcers in diabetic Charcot feet. J Wound Care 2001;10:323–8.
8. Sohn MW, Stuck RM, Pinzur M, et al. Lower-extremity amputation risk after Charcot arthropathy and diabetic foot ulcer. Diabetes Care 2010;33:98–100.
9. Petrova NL, Edmonds ME. Charcot neuro-osteoarthropathy-current standards. Diabetes Metab Res Rev 2008;24(Suppl 1):S58–61.
10. Katoulis EC, Ebdon-Parry M, Lanshammar H, et al. Gait abnormalities in diabetic neuropathy. Diabetes Care 1997;20:1904–7.
11. Armstrong DG, Todd WF, Lavery LA, et al. The natural history of acute Charcot's arthropathy in a diabetic foot specialty clinic. Diabet Med 1997;14:357–63.
12. Valabhji J. Immunosuppression therapy posttransplantation can be associated with a different clinical phenotype for diabetic Charcot foot neuroarthropathy. Diabetes Care 2011;34:e135.
13. Rogers LC, Frykberg RG, Armstrong DG, et al. The Charcot foot in diabetes. Diabetes Care 2011;34:2123–9.
14. Ertugrul BM, Lipsky BA, Savk O. Osteomyelitis or Charcot neuro-osteoarthropathy? Differentiating these disorders in diabetic patients with a foot problem. Diabet Foot Ankle 2013;4. http://dx.doi.org/10.3402/dfa.v4i0.21855.
15. Petrova NL, Moniz C, Elias DA, et al. Is there a systemic inflammatory response in the acute Charcot foot? Diabetes Care 2007;30:997–8.
16. Sanders LJ, Frykberg RG. Charcot neuroarthropathy of the foot. In: Bowker JH, Phiefer MA, editors. Levin & O'Neal's the diabetic foot. 6th edition. St Louis (MO): Mosby; 2001. p. 439–66.
17. Chantelau EA. Start treatment early to avoid Charcot foot deformity. BMJ 2012; 344:e2765.
18. Chantelau E. The perils of procrastination: effects of early vs. delayed detection and treatment of incipient Charcot fracture. Diabet Med 2005;22:1707–12.
19. Sinacore DR. Acute Charcot arthropathy in patients with diabetes mellitus: healing times by foot location. J Diabet Complications 1998;12:287–93.
20. Pinzur MS, Shields N, Trepman E, et al. Current practice patterns in the treatment of Charcot foot. Foot Ankle Int 2000;21:916–20.
21. Game FL, Catlow R, Jones GR, et al. Audit of acute Charcot's disease in the UK: the CDUK study. Diabetologia 2012;55:32–5.
22. Bates M, Jemmott T, Moris V, et al. Total contact casting - a safe treatment modality in the management of Charcot osteoarthropathy and neuropathic foot ulcer. Diabet Med 2015;32:149.
23. Wukich DK, Motko J. Safety of total contact casting in high-risk patients with neuropathic foot ulcers. Foot Ankle Int 2004;25:556–60.
24. Pinzur MS, Lio T, Posner M. Treatment of Eichenholtz stage I Charcot foot arthropathy with a weightbearing total contact cast. Foot Ankle Int 2006;27:324–9.
25. de Souza LJ. Charcot arthropathy and immobilization in a weight-bearing total contact cast. J Bone Joint Surg Am 2008;90:754–9.
26. Petrova NL, Dew TK, Musto RL, et al. Inflammatory and bone turnover markers in a cross-sectional and prospective study of acute Charcot osteoarthropathy. Diabet Med 2015;32:267–73.
27. Folestad A, Alund M, Asteberg S, et al. Offloading treatment is linked to activation of proinflammatory cytokines and start of bone repair and remodeling in Charcot arthropathy patients. J Foot Ankle Res 2015;8:72.
28. Uccioli L, Sinistro A, Almerighi C, et al. Proinflammatory modulation of the surface and cytokine phenotype of monocytes in patients with acute Charcot foot. Diabetes Care 2010;33:350–5.

29. Armstrong DG, Lavery LA. Monitoring healing of acute Charcot's arthropathy with infrared dermal thermometry. J Rehabil R D 1997;34:317–21.
30. McCrory JL, Morag E, Norkitis AJ, et al. Healing of Charcot fractures: skin temperature and radiographic correlates. Foot 1998;8:158–65.
31. Moura-Neto A, Fernandes TD, Zantut-Wittmann DE, et al. Charcot foot: skin temperature as a good clinical parameter for predicting disease outcome. Diabetes Res Clin Pract 2012;96:e11–4.
32. Wu T, Chen PY, Chen CH, et al. Doppler spectrum analysis: a potentially useful diagnostic tool for planning the treatment of patients with Charcot arthropathy of the foot? J Bone Joint Surg Br 2012;94:344–7.
33. Hastings MK, Johnson JE, Strube MJ, et al. Progression of foot deformity in Charcot neuropathic osteoarthropathy. J Bone Joint Surg Am 2013;95:1206–13.
34. Zampa V, Bargellini I, Rizzo L, et al. Role of dynamic MRI in the follow up of acute Charcot foot in patients with diabetes mellitus. Skeletal Radiol 2011;40:991–9.
35. Chantelau E, Poll LW. Evaluation of the diabetic Charcot foot by MR imaging or plain radiography–an observational study. Exp Clin Endocrinol Diabetes 2006; 114:428–31.
36. La Fontaine J, Lavery L, Jude E. Current concepts of Charcot foot in diabetic patients. Foot (Edinb) 2016;26:7–14.
37. Petrova NL, Edmonds ME. Medical management of Charcot arthropathy. Diabetes Obes Metab 2013;15:193–7.
38. Petrova NL, Edmonds ME. Acute Charcot osteo-neuro-arthropathy. Diabetes Metab Res Rev 2015;32(Suppl 1):281–6.
39. Richard JL, Almasri M, Schuldiner S. Treatment of acute Charcot foot with bisphosphonates: a systematic review of the literature. Diabetologia 2012;55: 1258–64.
40. Gough A, Abraha H, Li F, et al. Measurement of markers of osteoclast and osteoblast activity in patients with acute and chronic diabetic Charcot neuroarthropathy. Diabet Med 1997;14:527–31.
41. Mabilleau G, Edmonds ME. Role of neuropathy on fracture healing in Charcot neuro-osteoarthropathy. J Musculoskelet Neuronal Interact 2010;10:84–91.
42. Jude EB, Selby PL, Burgess J, et al. Bisphosphonates in the treatment of Charcot neuroarthropathy: a double-blind randomised controlled trial. Diabetologia 2001; 44:2032–7.
43. Pakarinen TK, Laine HJ, Maenpaa H, et al. The effect of zoledronic acid on the clinical resolution of Charcot neuroarthropathy: a pilot randomized controlled trial. Diabetes Care 2011;34:1514–6.
44. Pitocco D, Ruotolo V, Caputo S, et al. Six-month treatment with alendronate in acute Charcot neuroarthropathy: a randomized controlled trial. Diabetes Care 2005;28:1214–5.
45. Bem R, Jirkovska A, Fejfarova V, et al. Intranasal calcitonin in the treatment of acute Charcot neuroosteoarthropathy: a randomized controlled trial. Diabetes Care 2006;29:1392–4.
46. Saiz E, Zimmermann EA, Lee JS, et al. Perspectives on the role of nanotechnology in bone tissue engineering. Dent Mater 2013;29:103–15.

An Overview of Internal and External Fixation Methods for the Diabetic Charcot Foot and Ankle

Crystal L. Ramanujam, DPM, MSc, Thomas Zgonis, DPM*

KEYWORDS

- Diabetic Charcot foot • Charcot neuroarthropathy • Diabetic neuropathy
- Internal fixation • External fixation • Reconstruction

KEY POINTS

- The ultimate goals for surgical reconstruction of the diabetic Charcot neuroarthropathy (DCN) foot and deformity are to avoid amputation and produce a functional lower extremity capable of weightbearing that has an intact soft tissue envelope and is free of infection.
- Considerations for methods of fixation may include bone quality, status of soft tissue envelope, presence of fractures and/or dislocations, prior surgeries, history of deep soft issue or osseous infection, ambulatory status, medical comorbidities, and body mass index of the patient.
- Internal fixation methods available for DCN of the foot and ankle include plantar plate application, intramedullary implants (solid or cannulated screws, nails, or rods), extramedullary implants (locking plates, fixed angle plates), or various combinations.
- External fixation for DCN of the foot and ankle includes circular, hybrid, and computer-based designs.

Surgical advances with regard to both techniques and devices have led to a wide range of fixation options for managing the diabetic Charcot neuroarthropathy (DCN) deformities of the foot and ankle. Choices include but are not limited to internal fixation (screws, plates, intramedullary nailing, or beaming), external fixation (circular, uniplane or biplane, hybrid, or computer-based constructs), and combinations of internal and external fixation. The literature is replete with cases detailing the use of these fixation

Disclosure: The authors have nothing to disclose. T. Zgonis is the Consulting Editor for the *Clinics in Podiatric Medicine and Surgery*.
Division of Podiatric Medicine and Surgery, Department of Orthopaedics, University of Texas Health Science Center San Antonio, 7703 Floyd Curl Drive, MSC 7776, San Antonio, TX 78229, USA
* Corresponding author.
E-mail address: zgonis@uthscsa.edu

Clin Podiatr Med Surg 34 (2017) 25–31
http://dx.doi.org/10.1016/j.cpm.2016.07.004 podiatric.theclinics.com

devices for correction of foot and ankle deformities caused by DCN; however, sound evidence for which techniques or devices are best for this patient population is yet to be determined. Because the clinical manifestations of this condition can be so variable, the surgical decision-making should be formulated based on each unique patient. The ultimate goals for DCN surgical reconstruction are to avoid amputation and produce a functional lower extremity capable of weightbearing that has an intact soft tissue envelope and is free of infection.[1] Choice of fixation can depend on many factors, including bone quality, status of soft tissue envelope, presence of bone defects and/or dislocations, prior surgeries, history of deep infection, ambulatory status, medical comorbidities, and body mass index of the patient.[2] Before embarking on any surgical reconstruction for DCN of the foot and ankle, proper perioperative considerations must be made to optimize the patient's healing. Treatment of this complex condition is highly specialized with a high risk of complications; therefore, knowledge of all available fixation methods is critical for best outcomes.

INTERNAL FIXATION FOR DIABETIC CHARCOT NEUROARTHROPATHY

Based on many mechanical failures in the early years of surgical reconstruction for DCN, it has become well-accepted that standard methods for internal fixation, including lag screws with plates, are usually insufficient to meet the demands of stabilizing DCN bone that is often weak, osteoporotic, and fragmented. This rationale has given way to the development and use of stronger approaches, including plates with locking and nonlocking capabilities, and intramedullary fixation via large screws, nails, or rods. Span, or bridge, plating a technique typically used in comminuted fractures, has been modified for use in DCN of the foot and ankle through the form of extended joint arthrodesis. In a case report, Capobianco and colleagues[2] demonstrated successful use of this technique in which the arthrodesis included adjacent joints in addition to the zone of injury to impart greater stability with reduced risk of further joint collapse (**Fig. 1**). Blade plate fixation is another method to provide stronger internal fixation that has been advocated for use in severe ankle and hindfoot deformities. This fixed angle construct was used by Cinar and colleagues[3] through a posterior approach for tibiocalcaneal arthrodesis in a small case series of DCN patients with positive results. Schon and colleagues[4] first popularized the concept of plantar plating, in which the plate is placed on the tension side of the joint for arthrodesis, reporting successful midfoot arthrodesis in 34 patients with DCN. They hypothesized mechanical advantages for this technique included improved strength of the overall construct and improved ability to achieve correction of the deformity.

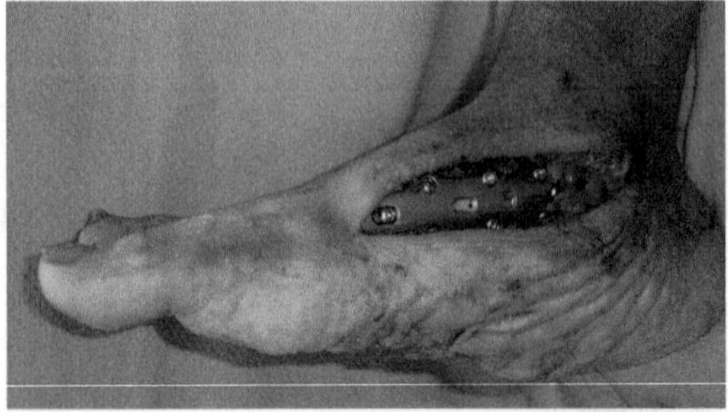

Fig. 1. Intraoperative internal fixation locking plating construct for extended medial column arthrodesis of the diabetic Charcot midfoot neuroarthropathy.

Intramedullary large diameter screws or rods have also been used in midfoot DCN through the technique of axial placement, or beaming, at the medial and/or lateral columns. The technique was initially described using cannulated screws; however, more recent reports have applied solid-core screws to impart increased strength to prevent loss of correction. Recent retrospective studies by Eschler and colleagues,[5] and Butt and colleagues,[6] have concluded that this implant should not be used as a stand-alone device but instead should be used with additional implants or constructs to allow healing and prevent failure. Intramedullary nailing is another method of internal fixation that has been used for arthrodesis procedures. This technique for ankle arthrodesis was first described by Adams[7] in 1948, although application of the device specifically in DCN of the ankle was not reported until Papa and colleagues[8] in 1993. Since then, larger retrospective studies, such as those by Pinzur and Kelikian,[9] and Dalla Paola and colleagues,[10] have demonstrated good fusion rates for DCN; however, those investigators also emphasized that other fixation methods, such as external fixation, should be considered in patients with large ulcerations. **Fig. 2** provides a diagram of internal fixation options.

EXTERNAL FIXATION FOR DIABETIC CHARCOT NEUROARTHROPATHY

External fixation for DCN of the foot and ankle has undergone a progressive and ongoing evolution. Generally, external fixation is described in categories including static, dynamic, or stabilization off-loading (**Figs. 3** and **4**).[1] Static external fixation, in the form of wire fixation and unilateral mini-external fixators, was initially reported by Sticha and colleagues[11] for DCN following corrective osteotomies and/or arthrodesis of the foot. In 2006, Pinzur[12] first described successful use of neutral ring external fixation to maintain alignment of deformity correction in 2 obese patients with DCN. Shortly thereafter, Pinzur[13] demonstrated the usefulness of circular external fixation

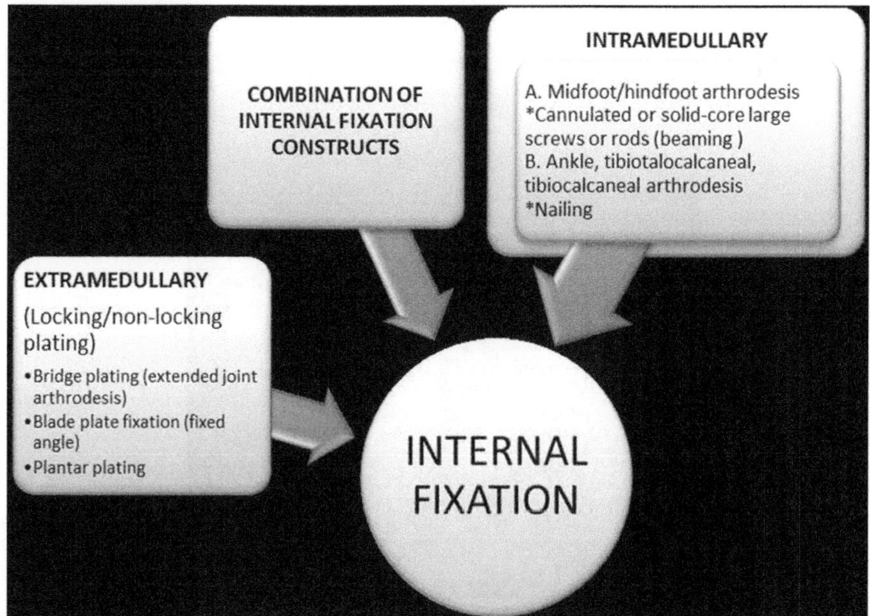

Fig. 2. Internal fixation for diabetic Charcot neuroarthropathy.

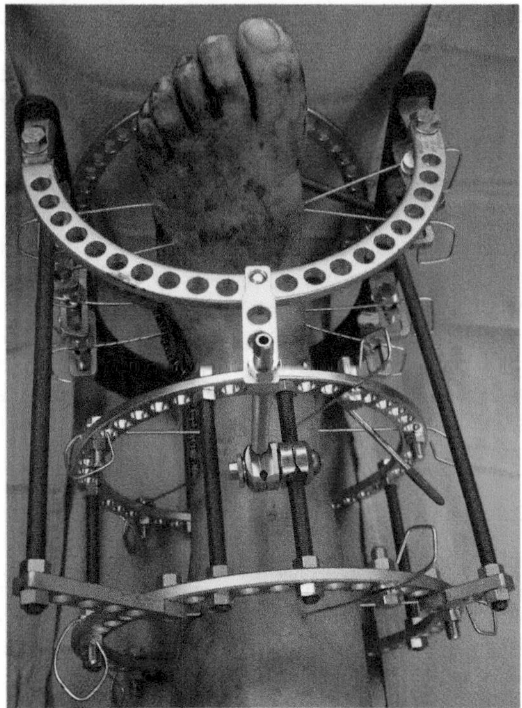

Fig. 3. Intraoperative static external fixation construct for ankle arthrodesis of the diabetic Charcot ankle neuroarthropathy.

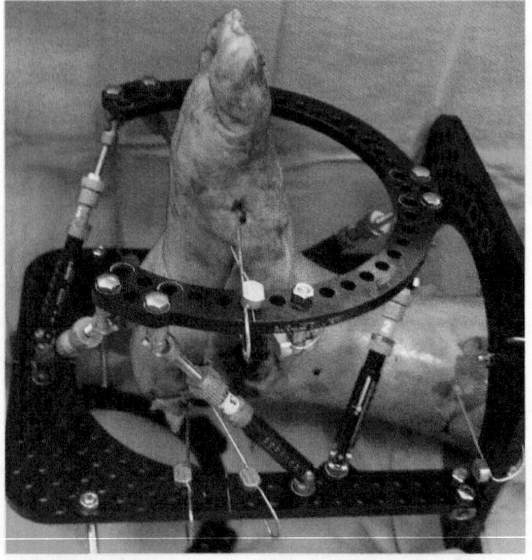

Fig. 4. Intraoperative clinical picture of a dynamic external fixation construction for surgical reconstruction of the diabetic Charcot foot neuroarthropathy.

for maintenance of operative deformity correction after resection of osteomyelitis in 14 DCN patients. In 2007, Lamm and Paley[14] reported the use of Ilizarov external fixation for gradual correction of deformity in severe DCN. These early reports highlight the benefits of external fixation for many possible challenging manifestations of DCN, including osteoporosis, decreased bone mineral density due to renal osteodystrophy, severe bone loss, postseptic deformity, prior or ongoing osteomyelitis, nonunion, peripheral vascular disease, and compromised soft tissue envelope.[1] Circular external fixation affords surgeons the ability to design a variety of different constructs to tackle deformity at multiple levels of the foot and ankle. In cases of severe deformity and dislocation with high risk of neurovascular and soft tissue compromise, gradual deformity correction can be performed using the traditional Ilizarov technique or dynamic external fixation constructs. Roukis and Zgonis[15] described the utility and technical demands of this computer-based system for dynamic correction of acute foot and ankle DCN. External fixation also allows for wounds to be addressed simultaneously in foot and ankle DCN, either with ongoing negative pressure wound therapy or with soft tissue reconstructive procedures such as grafts or flaps. Off-loading circular external fixation provides stabilization and continued access for local wound care to ensure success of such procedures.[16] Appropriate postoperative care of circular external fixation is imperative because complications, such as pin or wire tract infection and breakage, are possible. **Fig. 5** provides a diagram of external fixation options.

COMBINED INTERNAL AND EXTERNAL FIXATION FOR DIABETIC CHARCOT NEUROARTHROPATHY

Internal and external fixation constructs each have their own advantages and disadvantages, yet the literature is inconclusive on which technique is most effective for DCN of the foot and ankle. Combined internal and external fixation has become more popular recently in attempts to provide solid fixation and deformity correction to more complex DCN patients. In 2015, Hegewald and colleagues[17] published a retrospective case series of 22 patients treated with combined internal and external

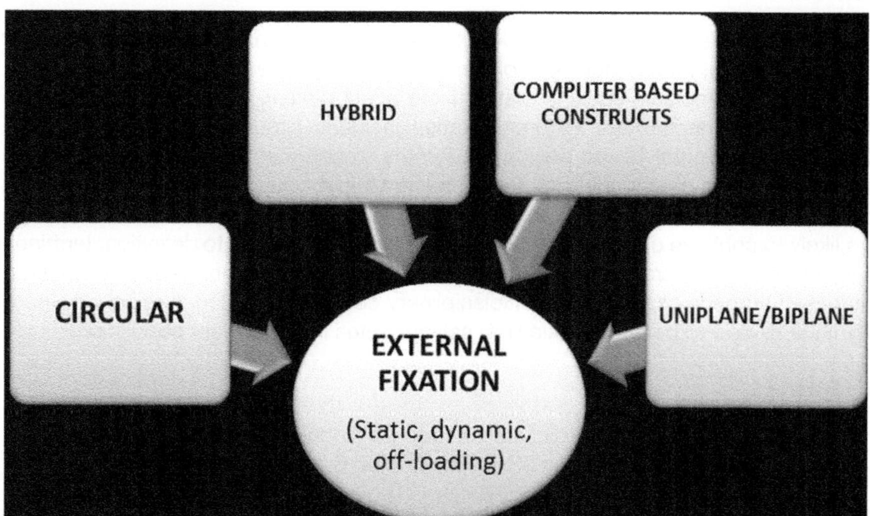

Fig. 5. External fixation for diabetic Charcot neuroarthropathy.

fixation for DCN, citing similar short-term limb salvage rates compared with either type of fixation alone; however, they pointed out the location of DCN varied in their study compared with others and this could impact the results.

Combined internal and external fixation methods may be used in the absence of ulcerations, septic arthritis, and/or osteomyelitis. Internal fixation is usually avoided in the presence of infection or even in cases of resected osteomyelitis, if feasible. However, in cases with a large osseous defect after resected bone for osteomyelitis, followed by local and systemic antibiosis with negative bone cultures and histopathology, internal fixation may be used for achieving stability and long-term anatomic alignment. External fixation alone, or as an adjunctive therapy to internal fixation for further compression, stabilization, and surgical off-loading, provides the surgeon with greater options when facing the complex DCN foot and ankle deformities. External fixation can be used in the presence of acute or chronic DCN ulcers, concomitant osteomyelitis, and also serves as a surgical off-loading device when plastic surgery techniques are used in the surgical reconstruction of DCN. External fixation can either be used in the form of a static or dynamic construct to provide acute or gradual correction in the DCN patient. Gradual correction may be used in the early phases of DCN by computer-based or traditional external fixation constructs. The theory behind the gradual correction concept for DCN is to allow for immediate correction and consolidation of the deformity while stabilizing and surgically offloading the affected lower extremity. Gradual correction may be followed by staged arthrodesis or stabilization procedures, and/or continuous off-loading and bracing postoperatively. Static external fixation constructs are typically used in the chronic phases of DCN, providing compression, stabilization, and surgical off-loading in major arthrodesis and/or adjunctive plastic reconstructive procedures. Static external fixation may also be used in the early phases of DCN when primary arthrodesis and consolidation of the deformity is indicated. Finally, hybrid external fixation, which combines circular and uniplane or biplane constructs, may also be used in DCN cases in which soft tissue reconstruction in large areas of the foot and/or ankle are also being performed, providing lower extremity stability and surgical off-loading.

SUMMARY

Internal fixation approaches available for DCN of the foot and ankle include plantar plate application, intramedullary implants (solid or cannulated screws, nails, or rods), extramedullary implants (locking plates, fixed angle plates), or various combinations of internal fixation devices. External fixation includes circular, uniplane or biplane, hybrid, and computer-based designs. Attempts to compare the methods of fixation are wrought with confounding factors, leading to inconclusive findings. The gaps in evidence-based medicine surrounding DCN foot and ankle surgical reconstruction are likely to continue unless a consensus is reached with regard to definition, terminology, classification, treatment indications, and operative techniques. Nonetheless, increased surgeon experience, multidisciplinary collaboration, and surgical advances continue to lead to better diabetic limb salvage rates in this patient population.

REFERENCES

1. Stapleton JJ, Zgonis T. Surgical reconstruction of the diabetic Charcot foot: internal, external or combined fixation? Clin Podiatr Med Surg 2012;29:425–33.
2. Capobianco CM, Stapleton JJ, Zgonis T. The role of an extended medial column arthrodesis for Charcot midfoot neuroarthropathy. Diabet Foot Ankle 2010;1. http://dx.doi.org/10.3402/dfa.v1i0.5282.

3. Cinar M, Derincek A, Akpinar S. Tibiocalcaneal arthrodesis with posterior blade plate in diabetic neuroarthropthy. Foot Ankle Int 2010;31:511–6.
4. Schon LC, Easley ME, Weinfeld SB. Charcot neuroarthropathy of the foot and ankle. Clin Orthop Relat Res 1998;349:116–31.
5. Eschler A, Wussow A, Ulmar B, et al. Intramedullary medial column support with the midfoot fusion bolt (MFB) is not sufficient for osseous healing of arthrodesis in neuroosteoarthropathic feet. Injury 2014;45:S38–43.
6. Butt DA, Hester T, Bilal A, et al. The medial column synthes midfoot fusion bolt is associated with unacceptable rates of failure in corrective fusion for Charcot deformity: results from a consecutive case series. Bone Joint J 2015;97:809–13.
7. Adams JC. Arthrodesis of the ankle joint: experiences with the transfibular approach. J Bone Joint Surg Br 1948;30:506–11.
8. Papa J, Myerson M, Girard P. Salvage with arthrodesis, in intractable diabetic neuropathic arthropathy of the foot and ankle. J Bone Joint Surg 1993;75:1056–66.
9. Pinzur MS, Kelikian A. Charcot ankle fusion with a retrograde locked intramedullary nail. Foot Ankle Int 1997;18:699–704.
10. Dalla Paola L, Volpe A, Varotto D, et al. Use of a retrograde nail for ankle arthrodesis in Charcot neuroarthropathy: a limb salvage procedure. Foot Ankle Int 2007;28:967–70.
11. Sticha RS, Frascone ST, Wertheimer SJ. Major arthrodesis in patients with neuropathic arthropathy. J Foot Ankle Surg 1996;35:560–6.
12. Pinzur MS. The role of ring external fixation in Charcot foot arthropathy. Foot Ankle Clin 2006;11:837–47.
13. Pinzur MS. Neutral ring fixation for high-risk nonplantigrade Charcot midfoot deformity. Foot Ankle Int 2007;28:961–6.
14. Lamm BM, Paley D. Charcot neuroarthropathy of the foot and ankle. In: Rozbruch SR, Ilizarov S, editors. Limb lengthening and reconstruction surgery. London: Informa Healthcare; 2007. p. 221–32.
15. Roukis TS, Zgonis T. The management of acute Charcot fracture-dislocations with the Taylor's spatial external fixation system. Clin Podiatr Med Surg 2006;23:467–83.
16. Ramanujam CL, Facaros Z, Zgonis T. External fixation for surgical off-loading of diabetic soft tissue reconstruction. Clin Podiatr Med Surg 2011;28:211–6.
17. Hegewald KW, Wilder ML, Chappell TM, et al. Combined internal and external fixation for diabetic Charcot reconstruction: a retrospective case series. J Foot Ankle Surg 2016;55(3):619–27.

Surgical Equinus Correction for the Diabetic Charcot Foot: What the Evidence Reveals

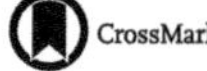

Claire M. Capobianco, DPM

KEYWORDS

- Equinus • Diabetic foot • Charcot neuroarthropathy • Achilles • Gastrocnemius
- Diabetic foot ulcer

KEY POINTS

- Ankle equinus is a known deforming force in the diabetic neuropathic foot and ankle.
- Surgery to address equinus in the diabetic and/or diabetic Charcot foot is often performed, but high-quality published evidence is scant and treatment guidelines remain undefined.
- Tendo-Achilles lengthening or gastrocnemius recession may be performed for addressing the underlying equinus deformity in the diabetic Charcot foot.

Triceps surae contracture, or equinus, is the lack of sufficient ankle dorsiflexion. In 1975, Sgarlato and colleagues[1] opined that 10° of dorsiflexion at the ankle with the knee extended is necessary for normal gait and less than 10° is considered pathologic. Although controversial,[2] these parameters are frequently used as endpoints in the literature. Equinus is correlated with upper motor neuron lesions as well as with local foot and ankle pathomechanics. Equinus is a significant deforming force that contributes to adult-acquired and pediatric flatfoot deformity, hallux abducto valgus, plantar fasciitis, Achilles tendinopathy, Charcot neuroarthropathy (CN), and plantar neuropathic ulcerations. Many of these conditions occur insidiously, and are a result of pathologic compensation of the foot because of the restricted ankle dorsiflexion. In neuropathic patients with diabetes mellitus, the direct effect of equinus as well as the indirect compensatory pathomechanical forces can propagate ulcer formation or CN because of increased plantar pressures or shear forces.

EQUINUS PREVALENCE

The prevalence of equinus in the general population has not been robustly studied. In the diabetic patient population, the reported prevalence of equinus ranges from

---

Disclosure: The author has nothing to disclose.

Orthopaedic Associates of Southern Delaware, 1539 Savannah Road, Suite 203, Lewes, DE 19958, USA
E-mail address: ccapobianco@delawarebonedocs.com

Clin Podiatr Med Surg 34 (2017) 33–41
http://dx.doi.org/10.1016/j.cpm.2016.07.005 podiatric.theclinics.com
0891-8422/17/

10% to 56%, and the variability is postulated to be secondary to inconsistent definitions of the condition.[3,4] Lavery and colleagues[3] evaluated 1666 consecutive patients with diabetes mellitus in an urban outpatient clinic and found a 10.3% prevalence of equinus. Additionally, these researchers, and others,[4] have noted a positive association between duration of diabetes mellitus and presence of equinus. In 2012, Frykberg and colleagues[5] undertook a prospective pilot study of 102 outpatients (43 diabetic, 59 nondiabetic) in a podiatric practice. Goniometric evaluation was used to evaluate for equinus, which they defined, narrowly, as ankle dorsiflexion of 0° or less. They found a prevalence of equinus in 24.5% of the population. Broken down, the diabetes cohort demonstrated a 37.2% prevalence of equinus and the nondiabetic cohort demonstrated a 15.3% prevalence of equinus, but this finding did not attain statistical significance. Based on history and additional clinical information, the researchers noted that equinus imparted a fourfold risk of ulceration in the diabetic cohort, and also noted a 2.8 times greater risk of equinus in patients with peripheral neuropathy. To date, no studies exclusively describe the prevalence of equinus in neuropathic diabetic patients with CN.

An additional paper by Hill[6] evaluated all new patients in his podiatric office and found that 176 out of 209 patients demonstrated restricted ankle dorsiflexion. Rao and colleagues[4] indicated that 12.5% of their control (nondiabetic) cohort and 56% of the diabetic cohort had less than 10° of dorsiflexion. Of note, this study specifically excluded neuropathic diabetic patients with ipsilateral or contralateral CN.

DIABETIC NEUROPATHY AND CHARCOT NEUROARTHROPATHY PREVALENCE

In the diabetic population, there is considerable variation in the published prevalence of neuropathy and CN. The European Diabetes Centers study of insulin-dependent diabetic patients (n = 3250) showed a prevalence of neuropathy in 28% of patients.[7] A study in Singapore in 2002 published a prevalence of neuropathy in 42% of the diabetic patients enrolled in the study, and a prevalence of CN in 2% of their patients.[8] The estimated prevalence of CN is under debate, with some researchers suggesting 1%[9] prevalence in all neuropathic patients and others suggesting up to 29% prevalence.[10,11]

CLINICAL EVALUATION OF EQUINUS

Evaluation techniques for equinus include the following

- Silfverskiold test: Have the patient seated, rotate the subtalar joint into neutral, dorsiflex the ankle, and look at the relationship of the heel/hindfoot to the leg. Have the patient flex their knee (to relax the gastrocnemius) and reexamine the hindfoot–leg relationship. If they cannot dorsiflex 10° past neutral in either case, this indicates gastrosoleal (or osseous) equinus. If they can dorsiflex 10° past neutral only with the knee flexed, this indicates gastrocnemius equinus. The interrater reliability of the Silfverskiold has been debated.
- The weight-bearing lunge test may be used in patients who are not at risk of falls. This method is primarily described in the physical therapy literature, but demonstrates good intrarater and interrater reliability.[12–14] The patient stands, facing a wall, with the foot pointed straight forward toward the wall, and the ipsilateral knee bent just so that the knee contacts the wall. Next, the patient slides the ipsilateral heel posteriorly (away from the wall) until the heel no longer contacts the ground. The distance between the wall and the longest toe, using an inclinometer

on the tibia, or using a goniometer between the fibula and the weight-bearing surface. The reported normal distance between wall and longest toe is 9 to 10 cm.
- Goniometery has long been used to quantify the degree of equinus, but this method is known to have poor interuser reliability.[15–18] Novel equinometers[19–21] have higher intrauser and interuser reliability and have been validated in the literature. This said, visual estimation remains the most frequently used assessment of equinus.

EFFECTS OF EQUINUS ON LOWER EXTREMITY BIOMECHANICS IN DIABETIC PATIENTS

A metaanalysis of 11 gait variables was performed in a systemic review of 16 biomechanical studies on patients with diabetes. In it, 382 diabetic neuropathic patients, 216 diabetic nonneuropathic patients, and 207 healthy controls were evaluated and the results indicated that patients with diabetic peripheral neuropathy have elevated plantar pressures and occupy a longer duration of time in the stance-phase during gait.[22] Lavery and colleagues,[3] in 2002, reported that a lack of dorsiflexion increases peak plantar pressures 3-fold. In a separate study of 164 diabetic patients, Armstrong and Lavery indicated that those with acute CN and those with neuropathic ulcerations had significantly higher peak plantar pressures compared with those who had neuropathy without ulceration, and those who were neurologically intact. These findings suggest that increased peak plantar pressures predispose the diabetic neuropathic patient to the potentially devastating sequelae of CN or ulceration.[23]

Decades before this systematic analysis, Ctercteko and colleagues[24] compared vertical forces acting on the feet of a small cohort of diabetic patients who had a neuropathic ulceration versus diabetic neuropathic patients without ulcer versus nondiabetic nonneuropathic nonulcerated patients. The researchers found that, independent of ulceration presence, the neuropathic groups transmitted less force through the toes and demonstrated medial shift of the weight-bearing force through the metatarsal heads. They also found that the absolute force was significantly greater in the ulcer cohort than in both control groups.[24]

GENERAL CONSIDERATIONS REGARDING TREATMENT OPTIONS FOR DIABETIC NEUROPATHIC PATIENTS WITH EQUINUS

Although the pathophysiology behind advance glycosylation endproducts is well-understood, scant basic science literature exists regarding the associated surgical ramifications of the molecular alterations in these tissues. Grant and colleagues[25] published an electron micrography-based study that examined 17 Achilles tendons (12 in diabetic patients with CN and/or ulcerations and 5 in nondiabetic patients). All of the patients were noted to have gastrosoleal equinus. Of the 17 patients, 13 were noted to have CN. Presence or absence of ulceration was not detailed. No specifics on the surgeries performed on any of the patients was listed other than "surgery to repair common severe foot abnormalities"[25] was performed in the nondiabetic group.

The results notably demonstrated increased packing density of collagen fibrils, decreased fibrillar diameter, and abnormal fibril morphology in the diabetic patients. Additionally, the collagen fibril fine structure was noted to be twisted, curved, overlapping, and disorganized in the diabetic patients (11 of 12), but noted to be normal and regular in the nondiabetic patients. The researchers hypothesized that the morphologic irregularities in the Achilles tendons of diabetic patients reflected an ultrastructural reorganization that may be related to a cumulative nonenzymatic glycosylation process and may effect tightening or shortening of the triceps surae. The researchers also hypothesized that diabetes mellitus, not neuropathy, was the underlying etiology of both the fine structural and ultrastructural permutations noted in the diabetic neuropathic tendons.[25] Of note, duration of diabetes mellitus (range, 1.5–38 years) was mentioned, but glycemic control of the patients was not mentioned in the study.

NONSURGICAL TREATMENT OPTIONS FOR EQUINUS

Controversy exists regarding the efficacy of nonsurgical treatment options for equinus in the nonspastic population,[26,27] and virtually no literature addresses this question in the diabetic population. A single case study (of a healthy nondiabetic subject) details the application of a neuroprosthetic device to decrease plantar forefoot pressure via functional electronic stimulation of the deep peroneal nerve at heel strike. These devices are typically used to assist dorsiflexion to treat dropfoot deformity, but this study proposes a secondary application in the high-risk diabetic neuropathic patient with equinus. The authors detail approximately 20% to 30% forefoot pressure reduction with this protocol, and indicate that surgical interventions offer equivalent forefoot pressure reduction. The authors foreshadow application in diabetic neuropathic patients with equinus, and publish their methodology for future clinical research.[28] Of note, no mention was made of the test subject's ankle joint range of motion, which may or may not be a confounding factor in further research.

In the physical therapy literature, Salsich and associates[29] compared ankle range of motion in diabetic patients with neuropathy and in age-matched controls. Although they had a small cohort (n = 17), they found significantly less dorsiflexion at the ankle in diabetic neuropaths than in controls (P<.001). The authors suggest diabetic neuropathic patients have “short,” but not “stiff” plantarflexory muscles based on decreased excursion capability parameters. As a result, the authors imply a functional change in diabetic neuropathic tendons and muscles that precludes the use of stretching to improve ankle dorsiflexion.

More recently, Rao and colleagues[4] published a study that confirmed the presence in diabetic patients of both increased passive ankle stiffness in the ankle plantarflexors and decreased ankle range of motion. The researchers also noted that glycemic control, as well as duration of diabetes, both affected the stiffness parameters. Of note, this study specifically excluded neuropathic diabetic patients with ipsilateral or contralateral CN.

SURGICAL TREATMENT OPTIONS FOR SOFT TISSUE EQUINUS

Multiple surgical options exist for lengthening the triceps surae complex, and selection depends ultimately on the patient's underlying pathology. For gastrosoleal equinus, the following options exist: Percutaneous triple hemisection (Hoke's procedure), open Z-lengthening, and Vulpius V–Y lengthening. External fixation has also been used for gradual tendo-Achilles lengthening, when combined with rigid osseous adjunctive procedures. For isolated gastrocnemius equinus, the Bauman, gastrocnemius intramuscular aponeurotic recession, Strayer, or tongue-in-groove procedures are options.

The percutaneous triple hemisection is the most commonly performed procedure for Achilles tendon lengthening in patients with gastrosoleal equinus. Level 1a evidence on the use of the triple hemisection was published by Mueller and colleagues[30] in the *Journal of Bone and Joint Surgery* in 2003. In it, the authors randomized a group of 64 neuropathic diabetic patients with less than 5° of ankle dorsiflexion and the presence of a forefoot ulcer into the following 2 treatment groups: total contact casting (TCC), or TCC with percutaneous tendo-Achilles hemisection. The patients were evaluated for ulcer healing and recurrence. Their data showed that the risk for ulcer recurrence in the surgery plus TCC group was 75% less at 7 months, and 52% less at 2 years compared with the TCC only group.[30]

Hastings and colleagues[31] evaluated the effects of Hoke hemisection tendo-Achilles lengthening on muscle function and gait in a case report of a patient with diabetes, neuropathy and recurrent forefoot ulcer. They found that tendo-Achilles lengthening improved ankle dorsiflexion, decreased peak plantar pressures and improved overall walking ability. In this case study, active or historical CN was noted to be in the exclusion criteria.

Less frequently used options for gastrosoleal equinus include the open Z-lengthening, the Vulpius V–Y lengthening, the transverse gastrosoleal recession, or in the most extreme cases, the complete Achilles tenotomy. The open Z-lengthening of the Achilles tendon offers the benefit of direct visualization and control of the amount of lengthening desired. The Vulpius V–Y advancement is not often used, but remains in the surgeon's armamentarium for lengthening.

For purely gastrocnemius equinus, the gastrocnemius aponeurosis is lengthened in either a transverse fashion or a tongue-in-groove fashion. Significant muscular weakening, poor cosmesis, and sural nerve proximity have been described with the tongue-in-groove techniques, so these have largely fallen out of favor. The transverse aponeurotic recession may be performed just distal to gastrocnemius muscle belly runout (Strayer procedure), just proximal to the gastrocnemius muscle belly runout (gastrocnemius intramuscular aponeurotic recession or "high Strayer" procedure), or with multiple adjacent transverse recessions performed intramuscularly, more proximally, and in succession (Bauman procedure). The advantages of the transverse-type recessions include better cosmesis, less postoperative muscle atrophy, and less neurovascular risk.

POTENTIAL COMPLICATIONS WITH SURGICAL EQUINUS TREATMENT

Specific surgical complications in this high-risk patient population simply include undercorrection and overcorrection. As a result of the anatomy of the Achilles tendon, the gastrocnemius recession causes less of an effect on the passive range of motion of the ankle, and has a higher risk for undercorrection of the equinus deformity.

One of the most feared complications of surgical treatment for gastrosoleal equinus is overlengthening or rupture of the Achilles tendon. An overlengthened (or absent) Achilles lever arm can perpetuate apropulsive calcaneal gait and precipitate a troublesome inferior calcaneal ulceration. In 2004, Holstein and colleagues[32] published a case series of 63 patients with neuropathic forefoot ulcers (total of 69 ulcerated feet), all of whom underwent percutaneous Hoke's hemisection Achilles tendon lengthenings. They reported an Achilles rupture rate of 10%, and noted that 47% of the patients with insensate heel pads developed transfer ulcers in the plantar heel. They also noted that 14% of the patients who had excessive dorsiflexion postoperatively (>15°) developed late heel ulcerations. Additionally, they noted an incidence of surgically induced postoperative CN in 4% of the patients. They concluded that loss of protective sensation of the heel pad increases the risk of transfer ulcers to the heel.

LITERATURE REVIEW

Sufficient data in the literature on equinus correction in CN are lacking. The surgical literature regarding CN in the foot and ankle almost exclusively details only osseous procedures, even though equinus is highly prevalent in this population and is universally accepted as the major deforming force in the neuropathic foot. Details regarding the definition of equinus used, measurement techniques used, and severity of underlying neuropathy are often completely absent from the methods, data, or discussion in surgical papers. In the few studies that mention adjunctive procedures for equinus correction, the explanation behind the surgical approach to the pathology is often omitted entirely.

Recently, Schneekloth and colleagues[33] published an updated systematic review of surgical management of CN in patients with diabetes, and noted that 30 reports, encompassing 860 patients, met the inclusion criteria for their study. Not a single procedure for equinus correction was mentioned.

Lamm and colleagues[34] mentioned the adjunctive equinus procedures during their CN reconstruction case series. They published a 2-stage percutaneous internal and external fixation approach to diabetic CN foot reconstruction on a case series of 11 feet in 8 patients. They noted that all of the patients had gastrosoleal equinus, and all of them underwent an adjunctive procedure for equinus. In the results section, the authors mention that gastrosoleal recession was performed in 3 patients and tendo-Achilles lengthening was performed in 8 patients. Confusingly, the statistical description of the case series notes that gastrocnemius recession (not gastrosoleal recession) was performed in those 3 patients. No techniques were discussed for the equinus procedures, and no equinometric data were provided or mentioned. They noted no complications specific to the equinus approach used, but did detail operative adjustments of external or internal fixation, 4 broken wires or half-pins, 2 broken rings, and 11 pin tract infections. The authors did specifically note the absence of recurrent ulcerations and the absence of subsequent amputation, with average follow-up of 22 months.

In 2005, Grant and colleagues[35] published a widely cited basic science paper that evaluated biomechanical characteristics of Achilles tendons in 20 patients with CN who were undergoing an open Z-lengthening of the tendon and compared these with 9 Achilles tendons from cadaveric specimens that were nondiabetic. They evaluated ultimate tensile strength and elasticity (via Young's modulus). The authors reported that the ultimate tensile strength at the break point was 2 times less in the CN tendons and also that Young's modulus (the slope of the elastic portion of the stress/strain curve) was 3 times less in the CN tendons. As a result, the authors concluded that a significant difference exists in ultimate tensile strength and elasticity between tendons of patients with CN foot and those of non-CN controls and that the Achilles tendon in patients with CN has significantly altered biomechanical properties versus normal tendons. This said, *P* values were not published, the graphs were inconsistent with the text in the article, and no mention was made of study shortcomings.

Clearly, no systematic reviews exist specifically regarding the surgical correction of equinus in CN feet. Only 1 systematic review exists regarding the entirety of surgical treatment of CN feet. In 2012, Lowery and colleagues[36] evaluated 95 articles (56% of which were retrospective case series and 44% of which were case reports) and excluded studies that had alternative etiologies for CN, were not written in English, and nonfoot/ankle or nonsurgical in nature. With these exclusions, 1143 patients were included in the systematic review. Of note, 4 centers contributed 51% of all patients reported. The authors noted that ancillary procedures (tendo-Achilles lengthening or gastrocnemius recession) were commonly used, but failed to detail the number or specifics of equinus procedures performed in the summary chart. The authors did offer a grade B recommendation for equinus correction in the CN foot.

SUMMARY

Consensus statements from professional associations[37] and Charcot task force committees[38] regarding the surgical treatment of equinus in patients with diabetes (with or without CN) are undefined. Evaluation of equinus in the diabetic lower extremity and diabetic CN examinations is cursorily listed only[37] and intramuscular lengthening of the gastrocnemius ought to be used in patients with insensate heel pads to avoid calcaneal gait and decrease the risk of heel ulcers in diabetic patients.[38]

As foot and ankle specialists, we concur that, surgical equinus correction is a critical part of our treatment algorithm, but equinus surgery in the diabetic CN is clearly not supported by fair evidence in the literature. Instead, the literature is replete with omitted information about these procedures in this population, and is often mentioned only in passing in the discussion. Caution should be exercised with tendo-Achilles lengthening or Achilles tenotomy in a patient with an insensate heel pad. In the specific population of profoundly neuropathic diabetic patients with anesthetic heel pads, selective gastrocnemius recession may provide satisfactory results.

Biomechanical studies have shown that ankle equinus significantly alters gait and plantar pressures, and in the diabetic neuropathic patient population, this can propagate plantar ulceration. Surgical correction of equinus is globally and frequently used to aid in plantar wound healing in the neuropathic diabetic patient, with and without CN. Additionally, more basic science research is needed on diabetic neuropathic Achilles tendons and published literature on CN reconstructive procedures needs to include more details regarding type of equinus correction performed.

REFERENCES

1. Sgarlato TE, Morgan J, Shane HS, et al. Tendo Achilles lengthening and its effect on foot disorders. J Am Podiatry Assoc 1975;65:849–71.
2. Charles J, Scutter SD, Buckley J. Static ankle joint equinus: toward a standard definition and diagnosis. J Am Podiatr Med Assoc 2010;100:195–203.
3. Lavery LA, Armstrong DG, Boulton AJ, et al. Ankle equinus deformity and its relationship to high plantar pressure in a large population with diabetes mellitus. J Am Podiatr Med Assoc 2002;92:479–82.
4. Rao SR, Saltzman CL, Wilken J, et al. Increased passive ankle stiffness and reduced dorsiflexion range of motion in individuals with diabetes mellitus. Foot Ankle Int 2006;27:617–22.
5. Frykberg RG, Bowen J, Hall J, et al. Prevalence of equinus in diabetic versus nondiabetic patients. J Am Podiatr Med Assoc 2012;102:84–8.
6. Hill RS. Ankle equinus. Prevalence and linkage to common foot pathology. J Am Podiatr Med Assoc 1995;85:295–300.
7. Tesfaye S, Stevens LK, Stephenson JM, et al. Prevalence of diabetic peripheral neuropathy and its relation to glycaemic control and potential risk factors: the EURODIAB IDDM Complications Study. Diabetologia 1996;39:1377–84.
8. Nather A, Bee CS, Huak C, et al. Epidemiology of diabetic foot problems and predictive factors for limb loss. J Diabetes Complications 2008;22:77–82.
9. Jeffcoate W. Charcot neuro-osteoarthropathy. Diabetes Metab Res Rev 2008; 24(Suppl 1):S62–5.
10. Chisholm KA, Gilchrist JM. The Charcot joint: a modern neurologic perspective. J Clin Neuromuscul Dis 2011;13:1–13.
11. Slater RA, Ramot Y, Buchs A, et al. The diabetic Charcot foot. Isr Med Assoc J 2004;6:280–3.
12. O'Shea S, Grafton K. The intra and inter-rater reliability of a modified weight-bearing lunge measure of ankle dorsiflexion. Man Ther 2013;18:264–8.

13. Munteanu SE, Strawhorn AB, Landorf KB, et al. A weightbearing technique for the measurement of ankle joint dorsiflexion with the knee extended is reliable. J Sci Med Sport 2009;12:54–9.
14. Bennell KL, Talbot RC, Wajswelner H, et al. Intra-rater and inter-rater reliability of a weight-bearing lunge measure of ankle dorsiflexion. Aust J Physiother 1998;44: 175–80.
15. Ball P, Johnson GR. Reliability of hindfoot goniometry when using a flexible electrogoniometer. Clin Biomech 1993;8:13–9.
16. Rome K. Ankle joint dorsiflexion measurement studies. A review of the literature. J Am Podiatr Med Assoc 1996;86:205–11.
17. Martin RL, McPoil TG. Reliability of ankle goniometric measurements: a literature review. J Am Podiatr Med Assoc 2005;95:564–72.
18. Van Gheluwe B, Kirby KA, Roosen P, et al. Reliability and accuracy of biomechanical measurements of the lower extremities. J Am Podiatr Med Assoc 2002;92: 317–26.
19. Wilken J, Rao S, Estin M, et al. A new device for assessing ankle dorsiflexion motion: reliability and validity. J Orthop Sports Phys Ther 2011;41:274–80.
20. Gatt A, Chockalingam N. Validity and reliability of a new ankle dorsiflexion measurement device. Prosthet Orthot Int 2013;37:289–97.
21. Wilken J, Saltzman C, Yack H. Reliability and validity of Iowa ankle range-of-motion device. J Orthop Sports Phys Ther 2004;34:A17–8.
22. Fernando M, Crowther R, Lazzarini P, et al. Biomechanical characteristics of peripheral diabetic neuropathy: a systematic review and meta-analysis of findings from the gait cycle, muscle activity and dynamic barefoot plantar pressure. Clin Biomech 2013;28:831–45.
23. Armstrong DG, Lavery LA. Elevated peak plantar pressures in patients who have Charcot arthropathy. J Bone Joint Surg Am 1998;80:365–9.
24. Ctercteko GC, Dhanendran M, Hutton WC, et al. Vertical forces acting on the feet of diabetic patients with neuropathic ulceration. Br J Surg 1981;68:608–14.
25. Grant WP, Sullivan R, Sonenshine DE, et al. Electron microscopic investigation of the effects of diabetes on the Achilles tendon. J Foot Ankle Surg 1997;36:272–8.
26. Macklin K, Healy A, Chockalingam N. The effect of calf muscle stretching exercises on ankle joint dorsiflexion and dynamic foot pressures, force and related temporal parameters. Foot (Edinb) 2012;22:10–7.
27. Radford JA, Burns J, Buchbinder R, et al. Does stretching increase ankle dorsiflexion range of motion? A systematic review. Br J Sports Med 2006;40:870–5.
28. Bharara M, Najafi B, Armstrong DG. Methodology for use of a neuroprosthetic to reduce plantar pressure: applications in patients with diabetic foot disease. J Diabetes Sci Technol 2012;6:222–4.
29. Salsich GB, Mueller MJ, Sahrmann SA. Passive ankle stiffness in subjects with diabetes and peripheral neuropathy versus an age-matched comparison group. Phys Ther 2000;80:352–62.
30. Mueller MJ, Sinacore DR, Hastings MK, et al. Effect of Achilles tendon lengthening on neuropathic plantar ulcers. J Bone Joint Surg Am 2003;85A:1436–45.
31. Hastings MK, Mueller MJ, Sinacore DR, et al. Effects of a tendo-Achilles lengthening procedure on muscle function and gait characteristics in a patient with diabetes mellitus. J Orthop Sports Phys Ther 2000;30:85–90.
32. Holstein P, Lohmann M, Bitsch M, et al. Achilles tendon lengthening, the panacea for plantar forefoot ulceration? Diabetes Metab Res Rev 2004;20(Suppl 1): S37–40.

33. Schneekloth BJ, Lowery NJ, Wukich DK. Charcot Neuroarthropathy in patients with diabetes: an updated systematic review of surgical management. J Foot Ankle Surg 2016;55:586–90.
34. Lamm BM, Gottlieb HD, Paley D. A two-stage percutaneous approach to Charcot diabetic foot reconstruction. J Foot Ankle Surg 2010;49:517–22.
35. Grant WP, Foreman EJ, Wilson AS, et al. Evaluation of Young's modulus in Achilles tendons with diabetic neuroarthropathy. J Am Podiatr Med Assoc 2005;95:242–6.
36. Lowery NJ, Woods JB, Armstrong DG, et al. Surgical management of Charcot neuroarthropathy of the foot and ankle: a systematic review. Foot Ankle Int 2012;33:113–21.
37. Frykberg RG, Zgonis T, Armstrong DG, et al. Diabetic foot disorders: a clinical practice guideline (2006 revision). J Foot Ankle Surg 2006;45:S1–66.
38. Koller A, Springfeld R, Engels G, et al. German-Austrian consensus on operative treatment of Charcot neuroarthropathy: a perspective by the Charcot task force of the German Association for Foot Surgery. Diabet Foot Ankle 2011;2. http://dx.doi.org/10.3402/dfa.v2i0.10207.

Surgical Treatment Options for the Diabetic Charcot Midfoot Deformity

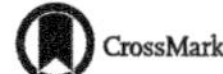

Yousef Alrashidi, MD[a,b], Thomas Hügle, MD, PhD[c], Martin Wiewiorski, MD[d], Mario Herrera-Perez, MD[e], Victor Valderrabano, MD, PhD[f,*]

KEYWORDS

- Charcot arthropathy • Diabetic Charcot foot • Charcot deformity
- Midfoot reconstruction • Cannulated screws • Chopart joint • Eichenholtz
- Diabetic foot

KEY POINTS

- Surgical treatment of diabetic Charcot foot aims at lowering its complications, including limb amputation.
- Charcot foot Eichenholtz stage III seems to be the right stage at which definitive reconstruction could be performed.
- Achilles lengthening or gastrocnemius-soleus release is an essential surgical step to lessen deforming forces and reduce recurrence rate of plantar ulcers.
- Understanding the concept of "superconstruct" can help surgeons to select the appropriate implants for diabetic Charcot neuroathropathy reconstruction.
- Reduction and fixation of the medial foot column is one of the keys of the successful surgical reconstruction of the midfoot.

Disclosure Statement: The authors have nothing to disclose.

[a] Orthopaedic Department, College of Medicine, Taibah University, PO Box 30001, Prince Naif Road, Almadinah Almunawwarah, Kingdom of Saudi Arabia; [b] Orthopaedic Department, Schmerzklinik Basel, Swiss Medical Network, Hirschgässlein 11-15, Basel 4010, Switzerland; [c] Rheumatology Department, Osteoarthritis Research Center Basel, Schmerzklinik Basel, Swiss Medical Network, Hirschgässlein 11-15, Basel 4010, Switzerland; [d] Department of Orthopaedic Surgery and Traumatology, Kantonsspital Winterthur, Brauerstrasse 15, Winterthur 8401, Switzerland; [e] Universidad de La Laguna, University Hospital of Canary Islands, Calle El Pilar 50 4 piso, Tenerife 38002, Spain; [f] Orthopaedic Department, Osteoarthritis Research Center Basel, Schmerzklinik Basel, Swiss Medical Network, Hirschgässlein 11-15, Basel 4010, Switzerland

* Corresponding author.

E-mail address: vvalderrabano@gsmn.ch

Clin Podiatr Med Surg 34 (2017) 43–51

http://dx.doi.org/10.1016/j.cpm.2016.07.006 podiatric.theclinics.com

INTRODUCTION

Progressive painless bony and articular destruction of the foot was first pointed out by Jean-Martin Charcot in 1868 in neuropathic patients with syphilis.[1] Later, Charcot arthropathy has become a description to any painless bony and joint destruction caused by longstanding neuropathy.[2] In particular, treatment of diabetic Charcot arthropathy of the foot (DCAF) is one the most challenging aspects in foot and ankle surgery.

DCAF may lead to deformity, ulceration, osteomyelitis, foot and ankle amputations, and limb loss and consequently interfere with patient's daily life activities and probably cause permanent disability. Severe DCAF with or without foot ulcer is a common reason of amputation worldwide. Thus, specific treatment protocols should be developed in order to provide a better care to DCAF patients to decrease the risk of amputation. Over many years, most published research work has been limited to level IV and V evidence-based medicine. Goals of treatment have been directed toward decreasing the rate of amputation through prevention of progression of foot ulcers (ie, through unloading of pressure sites), maintaining a stable plantigrade foot, and maintaining mobility of patients (ie, through avoiding prolonged immobilisation).

The Eichenholtz classification is still very useful in radiographic identification of the main sequential changes (stage I: stage of development and destruction; stage II: stage of coalescence and repair; and stage III: stage of consolidation and ankylosis).[3] Stage 0 Eichenholtz was proposed later to represent the presence of swelling, warmth, and instability without detectable radiographic changes.[4]

The Brodsky classification system is used to stage the DCAF depending on the anatomic location and extent of disease.[5] Type 1 (70% of cases) demonstrates the involvement of the midfoot (metatarsocuneiform and naviculocuneiform joints). Type 2 (about 20% of cases) demonstrates involvement of the hindfoot (subtalar [ST], talonavicular [TN], or calcaneocuboid [CC] joints). Type 3 (about 10% of cases) demonstrates involvement of the ankle joint (type 3A) and posterior calcaneus (type 3B). Type 2 likely presents with a rocker-bottom foot with development of symptomatic plantar ulcerations and associated bony lesions. Type 2 and type 3 may lead to foot instability. Surgical reconstruction in DCAF is technically challenging. This review article discusses a surgical treatment strategy for DCAF, which represents mainly the senior author's (V.V.) experience.

SURGICAL TREATMENT OPTIONS

Treatment of Eichenholtz stages I and II is usually conservative with bracing, total contact cast, and/or weight-bearing protection.[6] Moreover, several clinical trials have examined the role of pharmacologic therapy (eg, bisphosphonates or calcitonin) in early stages of Charcot neuroarthropathy, and some showed its effectiveness in pain relief, bone mineral density enhancement, and helping in lowering progression of early Charcot neuroarthropathy.[7–9] However, a recent systematic review study has suggested that available evidence (including randomized clinical trials) does not support its routine use. Temporary external fixation is indicated in cases of foot instability or inability to brace the limb in cases of Eichenholtz stages I and II; presence of an active foot ulcer; or presence of osteomyelitis. External fixation is kept until reaching stage III and recovery from ulcers and infection (if present). Surgery is contraindicated in vascular insufficiency cases or nonsalvageable limbs.

Local or systemic infection has to be treated properly before proceeding to surgical reconstruction. MRI can be misleading because osseous changes of noninfected

Charcot arthropathy can be indistinguishable from osteomyelitis. Therefore, osteomyelitis should never be diagnosed by MRI alone because high false positive findings may lead to unnecessary medical and surgical interventions, including amputation.[10] Definitive diagnosis of osteomyelitis is made by bone biopsy in addition to clinical, laboratory, and radiological assessment. Osteomyelitis associated with DCAF should be treated aggressively in the form of debridement, temporary external fixation, and therapeutic antibiotics. Application of external fixators carries the risk of pin tract infection in these clinical case scenarios.

If reconstruction is attempted in Eichenholtz stages I and II, the bone stock may not be amenable to fixation with an increased chance of loss of fixation and infection. Despite lack of comparative studies on the proper timing of surgical reconstruction, Eichenholtz stage III seems to be the right stage for definitive foot reconstruction, which is characterized clinically by osseous stability and resolution of edema and erythema, and radiologically by osseous union.[5]

SURGICAL RECONSTRUCTION OF EICHENHOLTZ STAGE III MIDFOOT DEFORMITY

Preoperative Preparation

Clinical examination is essential to determine the soft tissue status, location of the greatest deformity, degree of bony instability (if present), and the vascularity of the limb. The hindfoot alignment preoperatively should be documented. It is important to delineate any involvement of hindfoot in DCAF because it has been observed that midfoot DCAF has a progressive tendency to involve the hindfoot, probably due to late diagnosis and late initiation of treatment.[11] Distal neurologic status should be documented (eg, examination of vibration, reflexes, or 2-point discrimination).

Depending on weight-bearing radiographs of the foot (triple view: dorsiplantar and lateral projection of the whole foot, anteroposterior ankle view, if available, hindfoot alignment view), the extent of joint involvement is assessed in addition to the quantification of amount of deformity (eg, talo-first metatarsal angle, TN coverage, varus/valgus alignment of hindfoot). Computed tomographic scan can be done in cases of severe deformities, wherein the surgeon may need to delineate the bony anatomy and defects.

Management of DCAF is a multidisciplinary team effort. The general condition of the patient and any associated comorbidities should be optimized. An internist or endocrinologist is involved to help in the care of glucose blood levels. The hemoglobin A1c level is a good long-term indicator of blood glucose control. To help check if the limb is sufficiently perfused, a vascular surgery specialist is consulted. Informed consent is taken for the surgical reconstruction with explanation of benefits and risks. Potential complications may include infection, nonhealing wounds, implant failure, nonunion, recurrent deformity, and amputation risk.[12]

Preparation of Joints

Careful and limited soft tissue handling by the use of less-traumatizing retractors is advisable throughout the surgical procedure. Adding to that, skin flaps are kept as full thickness as possible. The authors prefer to use a dorsomedial incision to approach the medial column, centered on the TN joint and a dorsolateral incision to approach the lateral column, centered on the CC joint.

Through the dorsomedial incision, the bony anatomy of the medial column is identified. TN, naviculocuneiform (Navcun), and first tarsometatarsal (TMT) joints are prepared using sharp curved osteotomes or chisels. Tibialis anterior tendon and neurovascular bundle have to be protected throughout the procedure. Through the dorsolateral incision, dissection is carried out carefully as the normal anatomy is disturbed and the cuboid bone may be found completely dislocated plantarly. A distractor or a spreader can be used to improve visualization and facilitate reduction of cuboid bone. If the cuboid bone is found dislocated, it is detached from plantar soft tissue, debrided, reshaped, and reduced to its anatomic position. Hypertrophied plantar soft tissue, which is a result of bony pressure, is preserved. Joint surfaces are refreshed and microdrilled. If ST joint arthrodesis is needed, preparation of the joint in a similar way through the posteromedial or posterolateral incisions or both. Osseous gaps are filled with allogenic (eg, bone chips) or autologous bone graft (eg, iliac crest graft). To enhance healing, it is advisable to use additionally orthobiologics, such as demineralized bone matrix, growth factors, or platelet-rich plasma.[13]

The authors recommend gastrocnemius-soleus release in significant midfoot Charcot deformity undergoing surgery to reduce dorsiflexion contracture, reduce the load on the sole of the foot, and reduce formation or recurrence of ulcers. In a systematic review with meta-analysis, Achilles lengthening or gastrocnemius release showed a lower rate of diabetic foot ulcer recurrence in comparison to total contact cast alone. The latter study suggests the effectiveness of Achilles or gastrocnemius procedures in management of the diabetic foot.[14]

Options of Fixation

To the authors' knowledge, there is not enough high level of evidence studies to support the superiority of a surgical reconstruction technique or a fixation construct over another in Charcot midfoot treatment. Use of solid screws, cannulated screws, conventional plates, locked plates, or a combination of plates and screws has been reported.[15]

For instance, fixation of midtarsal joints (TN and CC joints) in a nonneuropathic foot, from a biomechanical perspective, may necessitate insertion of at least 3 screws or a combination of plates and screws to overcome the expected high torsional forces across the joint. Appreciating added pathologic process in the neuropathic foot makes the surgeon realize the need for more efficient fixation constructs. Good rotational stability may significantly reduce chances of implant failure and infection.[16]

Understanding the concept of a "superconstruct" helps the surgeon in selection of the appropriate fixation construct depending on the patient's factors, such as soft tissue condition, bone stock, the need for bone grafting, and the severity of deformity (**Box 1**). Superconstructs may include the utilization of axial rigid screws encompassing healthy nearby joints, bridging locked plates, and/or plantar plates.[10]

Box 1
Factors that are considered in defining a "superconstruct"

1. Arthrodesis is extended beyond the pathologic zone to involve healthy joints.
2. Bone resection is carried out to shorten the limb, allowing for adequate deformity reduction without affecting the soft tissue coverage tension.
3. The use of strongest construct that can be tolerated by the surrounding soft tissue envelope.
4. The use of constructs that can be placed in a position that allows for maximal mechanical function.

Data from Sammarco VJ. Superconstructs in the treatment of Charcot foot deformity: plantar plating, locked plating, and axial screw fixation. Foot Ankle Clin 2009;14:393–407.

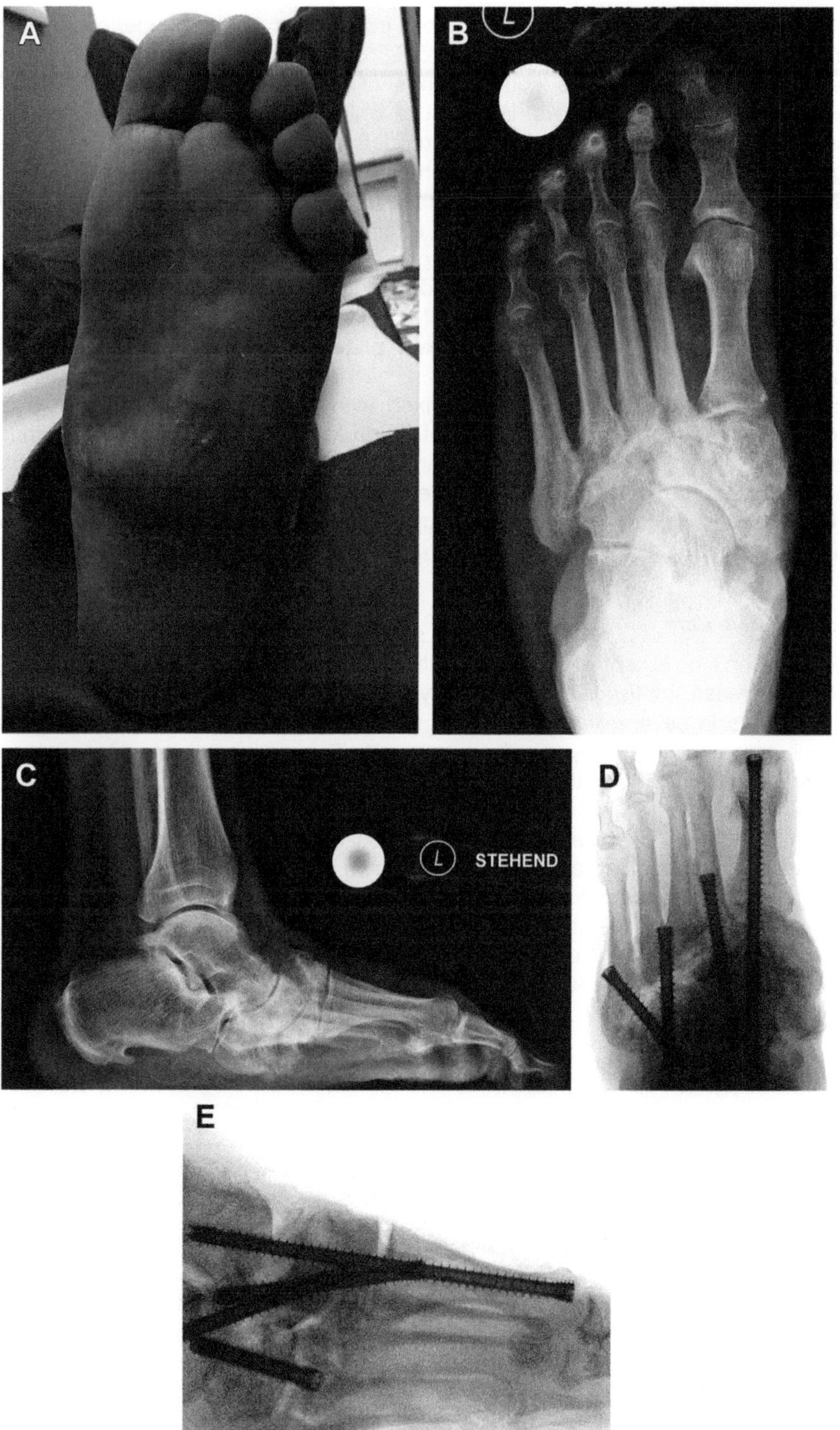

Fig. 1. Midfoot Charcot foot reconstruction. A 67-year-old man with longstanding diabetes mellitus presented to the clinic with midfoot Charcot deformity, Eichenholtz III. (*A*) Note the

The use of a single screw to fix the medial column carries the danger of breakage but has the advantage of fewer skin problems. Screw migration, loosening, and breakage were reported as complications of solid midfoot fusion bolt.[16–19] In contrast to cannulated screws, insertion of solid screws may be technically time consuming and has the risk of loss of reduction. The use of plates may have a higher chance of skin and soft tissue complications. The key to a successful midfoot deformity reconstruction is the reduction of the medial column. Provisional fixation of the medial column by the use of Kirschner wire is done first. Then, fixation is done by a retrograde cannulated compression screw (CCS; 7.0 screws, Medartis, Basel, Switzerland), which is inserted through the first metatarsal bone (MTB) head passing until the talus. The head of first MTB is approached through a small posteromedial incision. A bridging locked plate can be used as an additional fixation.

The cuboid bone is reduced and is fixed with retrograde cannulated CCS 5.0 screws, which are inserted in the base of fourth MTB or fifth MTB passing through the CC joint. Insertion of more than a screw passing through CC joint may not be possible due to reduced bone quality. If the ST joint requires fusion, the authors prefer to use 2 retrograde cannulated CCS 7.0 screws. A case of DCAF and its management is illustrated in **Fig. 1**.

Postoperative Care

The operated limb is kept elevated above the level of the heart during the first few days to help decrease soft tissue edema. Prophylactic intravenous antibiotics are continued for 48 hours in severe diabetic Charcot foot reconstruction. Pharmacologic deep venous thrombosis prophylaxis is prescribed. The peripheral vascular status is checked regularly. Physiotherapy in the form of lymphatic drainage exercises is started after the removal of stitches (usually 2 weeks after the procedure), and regular stretching Achilles exercises are recommended to prevent contracture recurrence. The authors prefer to use an orthosis that allows offloading the foot and ankle joint by transfer of the load from the knee joint to the ground (**Fig. 2**). The patient is mobilized strictly non-weight-bearing for at least 3 months, on crutches or with a special 4-wheel walker. An example of a convenient walker is shown in **Fig. 3**. Routine radiographs are taken at 6 weeks, 3 months, and every 6 months until there is clear evidence of fusion.

hypertrophic skin at the medial sole of the foot and absence of ulcers. Hypertrophic soft tissue resulted from longstanding bony pressure. (*B*) A preoperative anteroposterior radiograph shows diffuse collapse, sclerosis, and degeneration over the TN, first TMT, Lisfranc, and CC joints. (*C*) A preoperative lateral radiograph, which shows diffuse osteopenia; severe talo-first MTB malalignment; plantarly dislocated degenerative cuboid bone; subluxated and degenerated naviculocunieform joint. The edges of involved joints and newly formed bone can be clearly defined, which indicates Eichenholtz stage III. (*D*) An intraoperative radiograph, which shows midfoot fixation with 4 cannulated headless screws (CCS; Medartis): the first screw (7.0 mm) was used to fix the medial column; the second screw (5.0 mm) was used to fix the second TMT and TN joint, and the third and fourth screws (5.0 mm) were used to fix CC joint with entry points just distal to the fourth and fifth TMT, respectively. (*E*) An intraoperative radiograph, which shows an acceptable talo-first MTB alignment and CC joint reduction.

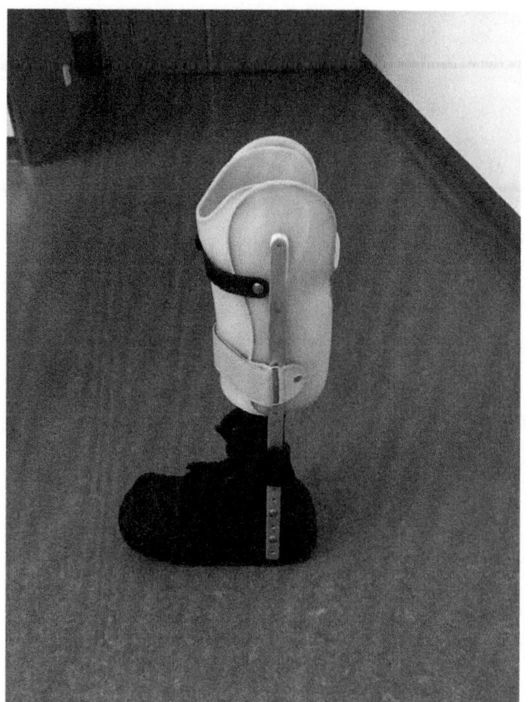

Fig. 2. An offloading orthosis.

SUMMARY

A suggested checklist for a successful diabetic Charcot midfoot Eichenholtz stage III reconstruction is summarized in **Box 2**. Future research must focus on well-designed prospective and controlled studies of diabetic midfoot Charcot reconstruction,

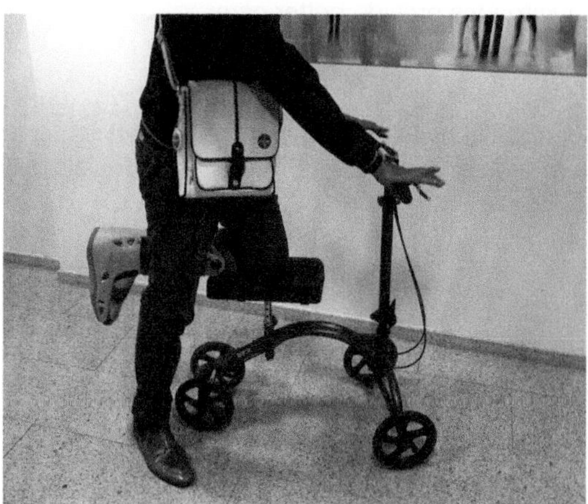

Fig. 3. A 4-wheel walker: a walker that resembles a scooter with a knee-supporting tray that allows good mobilization of the patient postoperatively without weight-bearing.

Box 2
Suggested checklist for a successful diabetic Charcot midfoot Eichenholtz stage III reconstruction

Preoperative

- HbA1c level
- Vascular consultation
- Bisphosphonates
- Vitamin D3

Intraoperative

- Prophylactic antibiotics
- Achilles/gastroc soleus release
- Restoration of the medial foot column
- Rigid fixation/superconstruct
- Bone grafting
- Orthobiologics

Postoperative

- Prophylactic antibiotics
- Strict non-weight-bearing (minimum of 3 months)
- Regular Achilles stretching exercises
- Bisphosphonates
- Vitamin D3
- Blood glucose control
- Minimizing edema (ie, lymphatic drainage, elevation)
- Special shoes after bone healing

specifically in terms of outcome and timing of surgical intervention, and establish clear guidelines that help surgeons provide better care.

REFERENCES

1. Charcot JM. Sur quelques arthropathies qui paraissent dépendre d'une lésion du cerveau ou de la moelle épinière [in French]. Arch Physiol Norn Pathol 1868;1: 161–78.
2. Jordan WR. Neuritic manifestations in diabetes mellitus. Arch Intern Med 1936; 57:307–66.
3. Eichenholtz CN. Charcot joints. Springfield (IL): Charles C. Thomas; 1966.
4. Shibata T, Tada K, Hashizume C. The results of arthrodesis of the ankle for leprotic neuroarthropathy. J Bone Joint Surg Am 1990;72:749–56.
5. Johnson JR, Klein SE, Brodsky JW. Diabetes. In: Coughlin MJ, Saltzman CL, Anderson RB, editors. Mann's surgery of the foot and ankle, 9. Philadelphia: Elsevier Saunders; 2014. p. 1397.
6. Pinzur MS, Lio T, Posner M. Treatment of Eichenholtz stage I Charcot foot arthropathy with a weightbearing total contact cast. Foot Ankle Int 2006;27:324–9.

7. Al-Nammari SS, Timothy T, Afsie S. A surgeon's guide to advances in the pharmacological management of acute Charcot neuroarthropathy. Foot Ankle Surg 2013; 19:212–7.
8. Pitocco D, Ruotolo V, Caputo S, et al. Six-month treatment with alendronate in acute Charcot neuroarthropathy: a randomized controlled trial. Diabetes Care 2005;28:1214–5.
9. Pakarinen TK, Laine HJ, Mäenpää H, et al. The effect of zoledronic acid on the clinical resolution of Charcot neuroarthropathy: a pilot randomized controlled trial. Diabetes Care 2011;34:1514–6.
10. Sammarco VJ. Superconstructs in the treatment of Charcot foot deformity: plantar plating, locked plating, and axial screw fixation. Foot Ankle Clin 2009;14: 393–407.
11. Ferreira RC, Gonçalez DH, Filho JMF, et al. Midfoot Charcot arthropathy on diabetic patients:complication of an epidemic disease. Rev Bras Ortop 2012;47: 616–25.
12. Wiewiorski M, Barg A, Hoerterer H, et al. Risk factors for wound complications in patients after elective orthopedic foot and ankle surgery. Foot Ankle Int 2015;36: 479–87.
13. Pinzur MS. Use of platelet-rich concentrate and bone marrow aspirate in high-risk patients with Charcot arthropathy of the foot. Foot Ankle Int 2009;30:124–7.
14. Dallimore SM, Kaminski MR. Tendon lengthening and fascia release for healing and preventing diabetic foot ulcers: a systematic review and meta-analysis. J Foot Ankle Res 2015;8:33.
15. Lowery NJ, Woods JB, Armstrong DG, et al. Surgical management of Charcot neuroarthropathy of the foot and ankle: a systematic review. Foot Ankle Int 2012;33:113–21.
16. Eschler A, Wussow A, Ulmar B, et al. Intramedullary medial column support with the Midfoot Fusion Bolt (MFB) is not sufficient for osseous healing of arthrodesis in neuroosteoarthropathic feet. Injury 2014;4(Suppl 1):S38–43.
17. Butt DA, Hester T, Bilal A, et al. The medial column Synthes Midfoot Fusion Bolt is associated with unacceptable rates of failure in corrective fusion for Charcot deformity: results from a consecutive case series. Bone Joint J 2015;97:809–13.
18. Richter M, Mittlmeier T, Rammelt S, et al. Intramedullary fixation in severe Charcot osteo-neuroarthropathy with foot deformity results in adequate correction without loss of correction—results from a multi-centre study. Foot Ankle Surg 2015;21: 269–76.
19. Wiewiorski M, Yasui T, Miska M, et al. Solid bolt fixation of the medial column in Charcot midfoot arthropathy. J Foot Ankle Surg 2013;52:88–94.

Surgical Treatment Options for the Diabetic Charcot Hindfoot and Ankle Deformity

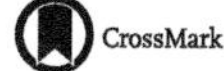

Tahir Ögüt, MD[a,*], Necip Selcuk Yontar, MD[b]

KEYWORDS

• Charcot • Ankle • Hindfoot • Surgery • Fixation • Diabetic neuropathy

KEY POINTS

- Charcot neuroarthropathy (CN) is associated with progressive, noninfectious, osteolysis-induced bone and joint destruction.
- Arthrodesis of the ankle and/or hindfoot is the method of choice when surgically correcting CN-related deformities in this region.
- Internal fixation, external fixation, or a combination of both can be used for the treatment.

Charcot neuroarthropathy (CN) is a progressive, noninfectious, inflammatory condition that leads to osteolysis-induced bone and joint destruction in patients with peripheral neuropathy.[1] CN has been associated with autonomic neuroarthropathy, infection (leprosy, human immunodeficiency virus), toxic exposure (ethanol, drug related), rheumatoid arthritis, multiple sclerosis, congenital neuropathy, traumatic injury, metabolic abnormalities, and syringomyelia.[2,3] However, diabetes mellitus has become the most common cause of CN in recent years. The incidence of CN is about 0.1% to 5% in diabetic neuropathy and is among the most fearful complications of diabetes mellitus.[4]

There are different types of classifications to describe CN that use clinical locations, radiological changes, and/or pattern of destruction. Eichenholtz[5] described the first classification system in 1966. His grading was mostly a radiological evolution of the condition; this was a source of criticism, but through time it is improved and supported with clinical manifestations.[1] Among the anatomic-based classifications, Brodsky[6]

Disclosure Statement: The authors have nothing to disclose.

[a] Department of Orthopaedics and Traumatology, Cerrahpasa Medical School, Istanbul University, Fatih, Istanbul 34098, Turkey; [b] Department of Orthopaedics and Traumatology, Istanbul Cerrahi Hospital, Hakkı Yeten Cad., Ferah Sok. No: 22, Fulya, Istanbul 34365, Turkey
* Corresponding author.
E-mail address: drtahirogut@gmail.com

Clin Podiatr Med Surg 34 (2017) 53–67
http://dx.doi.org/10.1016/j.cpm.2016.07.007

and Sanders-Frykberg[7] classifications include the entire foot and ankle, whereas Schon's classification[8] focuses on the midtarsus alone.

The Brodsky classification is based on 4 anatomic areas that are affected by the disease process. Type 1 is the most common form and constitutes about 60% of the Charcot feet. It involves all midfoot or portions of it. Type II has the main changes within the hindfoot and accounts for 30% to 35% of the Charcot feet. Type III has 2 subdivisions. Type IIIA has the changes within the ankle joint. When ankle involvement occurs, the talus is typically involved with fracture and fragmentation, leading to a nonsalvageable tibiotalar (TT) joint.[9] Type IIIB involves a pathologic fracture of the tuberosity of the calcaneus. Late deformity in this group of patients results in distal foot changes or proximal migration of the tuberosity that can lead to ulcerations and complicated with osteomyelitis. Type IV involves a combination of areas, and type V occurs solely within the forefoot.[10] For the purposes of this article, the management of Brodsky type II and III CN, which involve hindfoot and the ankle joint (**Fig. 1**), are discussed.

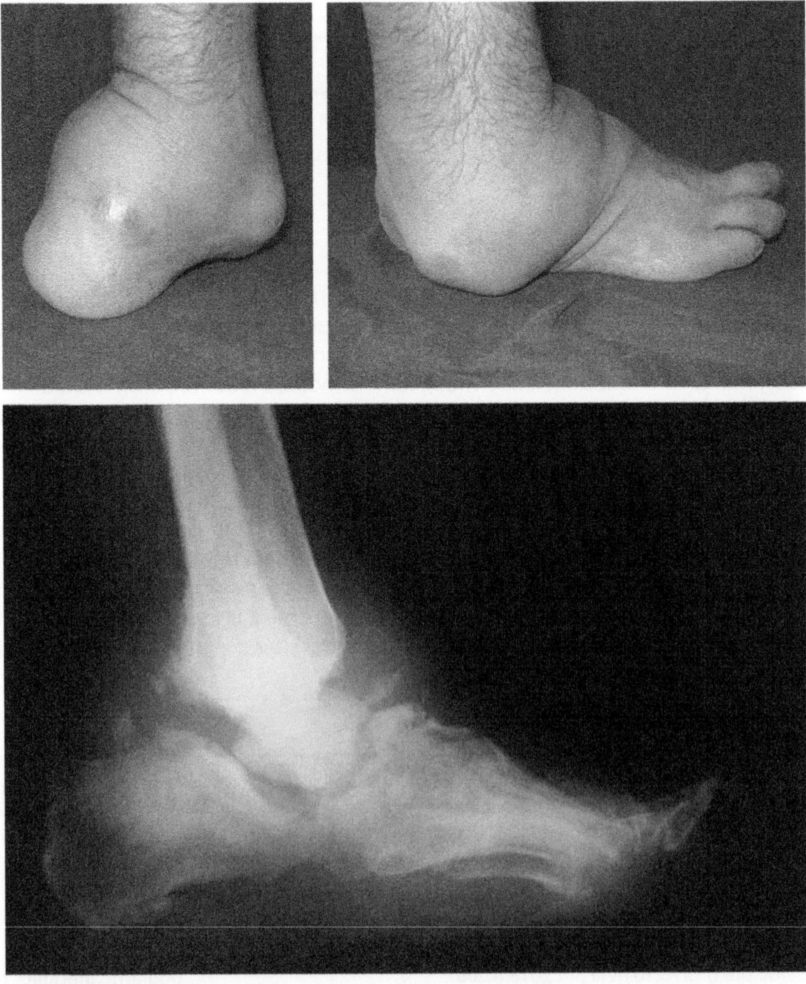

Fig. 1. A 57-year-old male patient with CN of the ankle joint.

Primary treatment of acute CN is usually nonoperative by using off-loading techniques such as total-contact casting (TCC) or various braces. Because Brodsky's type II and III are characterized by persistent skeletal instability, their conservative treatment may require longer periods of immobilization until Eichenholtz stage II and III are reached.[11,12] Although braces or TCC can be used in the treatment, prominent malleoli makes it difficult to brace deformities of the ankle and hindfoot. When there is significant deformity and instability that cannot be controlled with careful bracing, when ulceration occurs or is inevitable, when there is associated osteomyelitis or pain, surgical management is warranted in CN.[11,13] The aim of surgical treatment is to control and correct the alignment, decrease the risk of ulcerations and/or allow healing of them, treat osteomyelitis, and eventually mobilize the patient with a stable and plantigrade extremity.[14,15] Surgical treatment options may include Achilles lengthening, exostectomy, arthrodesis, and primary amputation.

ACHILLES LENGTHENING

Equinus contracture of the Achilles tendon is one of the most common deformities that is seen with CN.[14] Contracted Achilles tendon not only increases plantar peak pressures in the forefoot, it also stresses adjacent joints, frequently causing them to collapse and develop into nonreducible deformities.[16,17] Because of this, Achilles tendon lengthening can be used in conjunction with CN-related arthrodesis procedures to improve alignment of the ankle and hindfoot to the midfoot and forefoot.[11,18]

A percutaneous technique with 3-stab incisions is often preferred but the procedure has been shown to have some risks like overlengthening, iatrogenic rupture of the tendon during the procedure, and late rupture after ambulation secondary to a weakened tendon. Overlengthening may result in calcaneal gait, which may also complicate the process with the development of heel ulceration. To avoid overlengthening, selective release of medial plantar fascia was described, and Kim and colleagues[19] reported a 67% healing rate of forefoot ulcerations and no complications with this technique. Holstein and colleagues[20] reported a 10% rupture rate after percutaneous Achilles tendon lengthening in 68 patients' 75 ulcerated neuropathic feet. There is risk of hematoma formation, infection, and potential amputation after Achilles rupture in diabetic patients; because repair of the tendon is not feasible and is not usually recommended in this patient population, Stapleton and colleagues[16] recommended to treat ruptures with an ankle or tibiotalocalcaneal (TTC) arthrodesis.

EXOSTECTOMY

Exostectomy is most effectively used for Brodsky type 1 deformities, which involve the tarsometatarsal joints.[21] Unlike the midfoot, exostectomy is rarely successful at the level of the ankle and hindfoot because of the underlying malalignment.[22] It can be used to permit healing of a chronic ulceration around malleoli, which is usually associated with a coronal plane deformity.[11] It is also useful to minimize the deformity and consolidation-related bulky appearance around the ankle.

ARTHRODESIS

Arthrodesis of the ankle and/or hindfoot is the method of choice when surgically correcting CN deformities in this region. The goal of the arthrodesis procedure is to realign the foot on the leg and convert the deformed foot and ankle to a plantigrade one that is now stable, braceable, and walkable.[11] A stable pseudoarthrosis or so-called fibrous ankylosis is also accepted as sufficient for a good functional outcome in this patient population.[15] Successful arthrodesis requires careful removal of all cartilage and debris, debridement to bleeding subchondral bone, meticulous fashioning of bone surfaces for contact, complete debridement of soft tissues, and stable fixation.[14,22] In this process, osteotomies may also be required to correct the alignment of the ankle and hindfoot.[23]

If the deformity is isolated to the subtalar joint and/or Chopart joints, triple arthrodesis can be the procedure of choice. However, ankle and hindfoot involvement further complicates with collapse and destruction of the talar body, which increases instability around the ankle.[15] Deformities involving the body of the talus and/or ankle are usually treated with a TTC or tibiocalcaneal (TC) arthrodesis depending on the involvement of the talus. Pantalar arthrodesis is another option in these patients; however, TTC or TC arthrodesis is more preferable because they permit some motion at the transverse tarsal joints and this motion allows a small amount of plantarflexion and dorsiflexion.[22]

The choice of fixation (ie, internal, external, or both) depends on several factors. Internal fixation is not recommended in cases with poor soft tissue envelope, active infection, severe deformity preventing acute correction, and poor bone quality.[24–27] It is generally preferred to combine internal and external fixation in patients with morbid obesity, when there is a high risk for fixation failure or a need for soft tissue protection.

There are several options for internal fixation in the hindfoot and ankle. If a triple arthrodesis is performed, fixation is usually performed with multiple screws, but one has to be careful with their usage because they may not achieve adequate fixation for the large forces that will be placed across the joint[28,29] (**Fig. 2**). For arthrodesis procedures that extend across the ankle joint, screws, intramedullary nail, external fixator, locked plates, blade plate, and a combination of internal and external fixations can be used.

Intramedullary Nailing

The retrograde intramedullary arthrodesis nail offers stable intramedullary fixation and load sharing, and because of its intramedullary location, it can resist large forces.[17,30] Because of these advantages, studies reporting correcting ankle deformities in CN are more likely to use intramedullary nails[31] (**Figs. 3–5**).

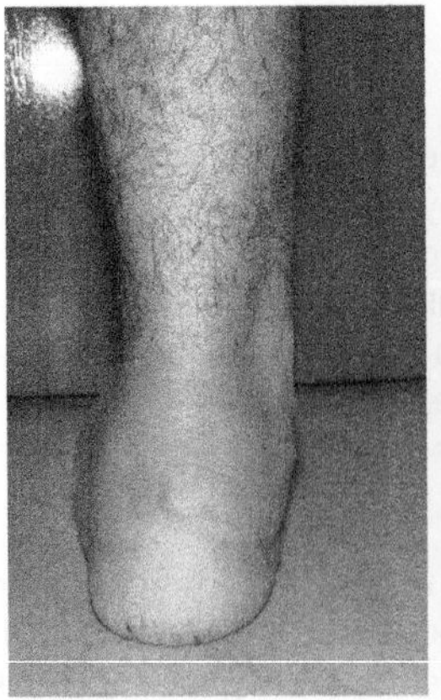

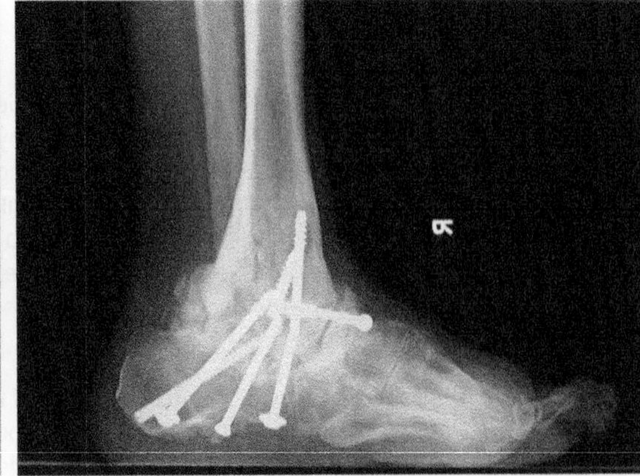

Fig. 2. Same patient as shown in **Fig. 1**, 2 years after surgery. Please note the stable and plantigrade weight-bearing foot achieved with multiple internal fixation screws.

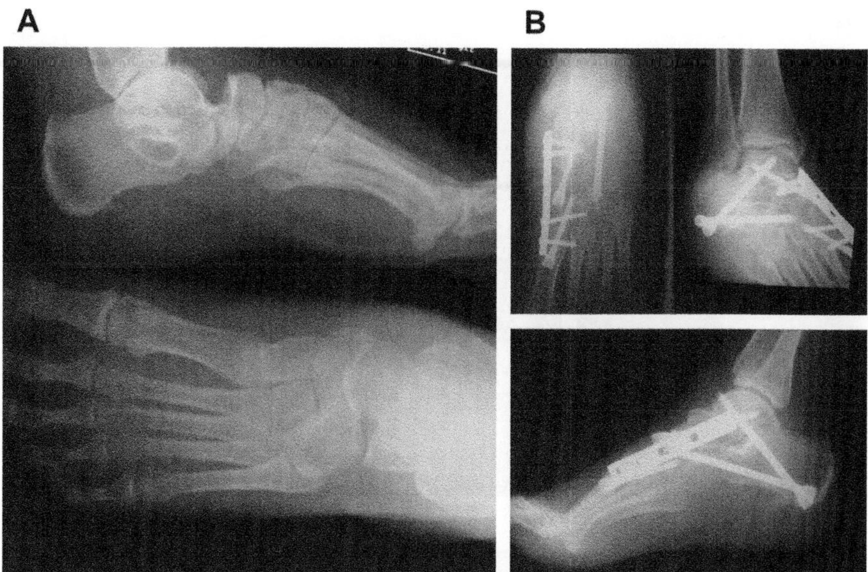

Fig. 3. A 51-year-old woman with neglected CN. Preoperative radiographs (*A*) show the deformity followed by a triple and first tarsometatarsal joint arthrodesis (*B*).

In 2006, Caravaggi and colleagues[32] reported results of 14 patients with CN involvement of the ankle and hindfoot. The investigators found that 10 patients (71.4%) achieved a solid ankle fusion, whereas 3 patients (21.4%) achieved a stable fibrous union that allowed ambulation in a brace. Three patients (21.4%) had hardware complications that necessitated removal, and one patient (7.2%) did eventually require a transtibial amputation for postoperative osteomyelitis.

Dalla Paola and colleagues[33] published the results of pantalar arthrodesis using an intramedullary nail in 18 patients with CN. Of the 18 cases, 14 resulted in stable union; the remaining 4 patients achieved a fibrous union. They did not observe any major complications, and along with satisfactory plantigrade positioning of the foot, limb salvage was accomplished in all 18 patients. Similarly, Siebachmeyer and colleagues[23] reported the outcomes of 20 patients' 21 feet with CN who underwent retrograde intramedullary nail arthrodesis. Limb salvage was achieved in all patients after a mean follow-up of 26 months and all patients except one regained independent mobilization in their study. One patient required revision surgery because of a broken nail, and they observed migration of distal locking screws when standard screws had been used but not with hydroxyapatite-coated screws (**Fig. 6**).

Recently, Ettinger and colleagues[15] published their results with surgical treatment of CN ankle involvement. Of the 58 patients, 38 were treated using intramedullary nail arthrodesis, 19 using an external fixator and 1 patient receiving neither. They achieved 100% fusion rate after intramedullary nail arthrodesis.

External Fixation

Although Farber and colleagues[34] and Pinzur[35] concluded that using external fixators leads to nonunion of TTC arthrodesis more frequently than does internal fixation, in cases of infection or poor soft tissue coverage, external fixation may be the only viable option. It is also biomechanically shown that in cases where internal fixation is not

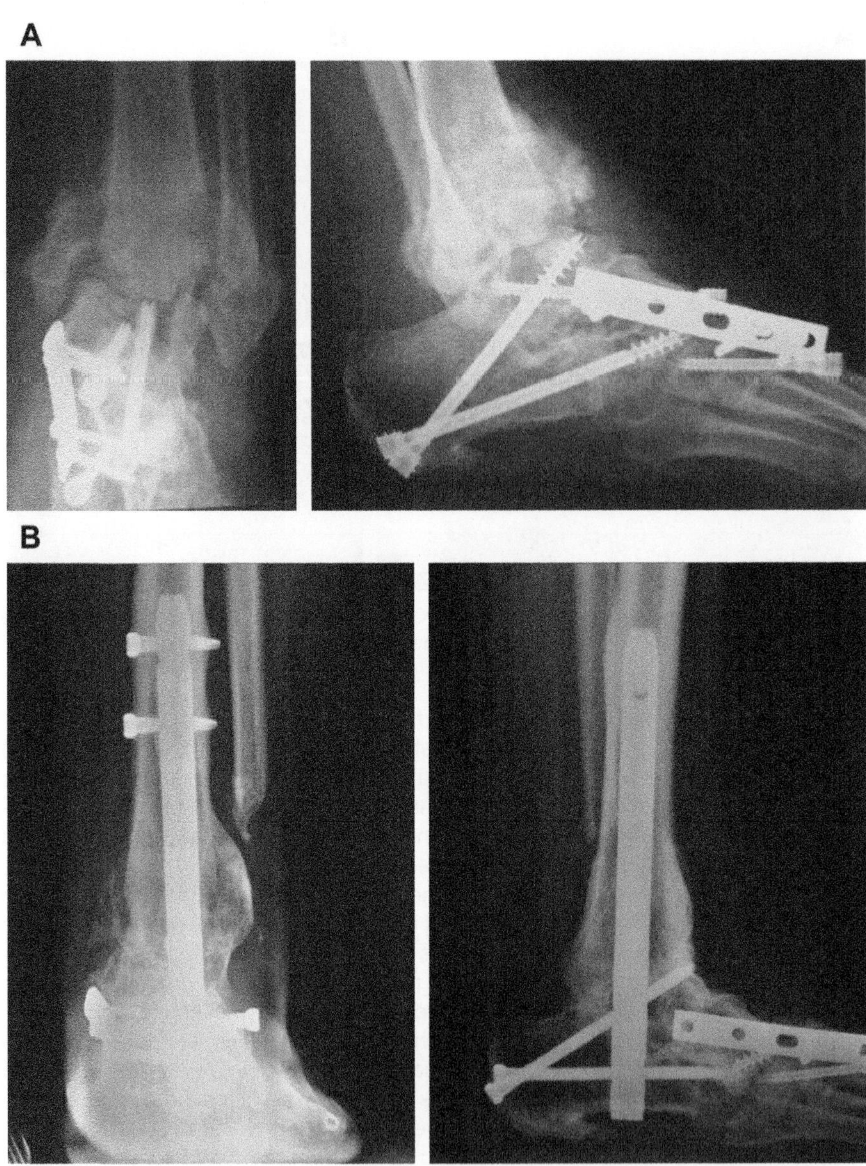

Fig. 4. Nine months after the original operation, the same patient as shown in **Fig. 3** developed CN in the ipsilateral ankle joint (*A*) followed by a TTC arthrodesis and intramedullary nailing (*B*).

appropriate, external ring fixation may be used with confidence.[36] External fixation also allows continued and immediate weight-bearing to patients who are not able to remain non–weight-bearing or in patients with a history or increased risk of deep venous thrombosis[9] (**Fig. 7**).

Fabrin and colleagues[37] evaluated the results of 12 ankles treated with external fixation for TT or TTC arthrodesis for CN with the presence of ulceration. They showed an overall salvage rate of 92% with only one leg requiring transtibial amputation due to

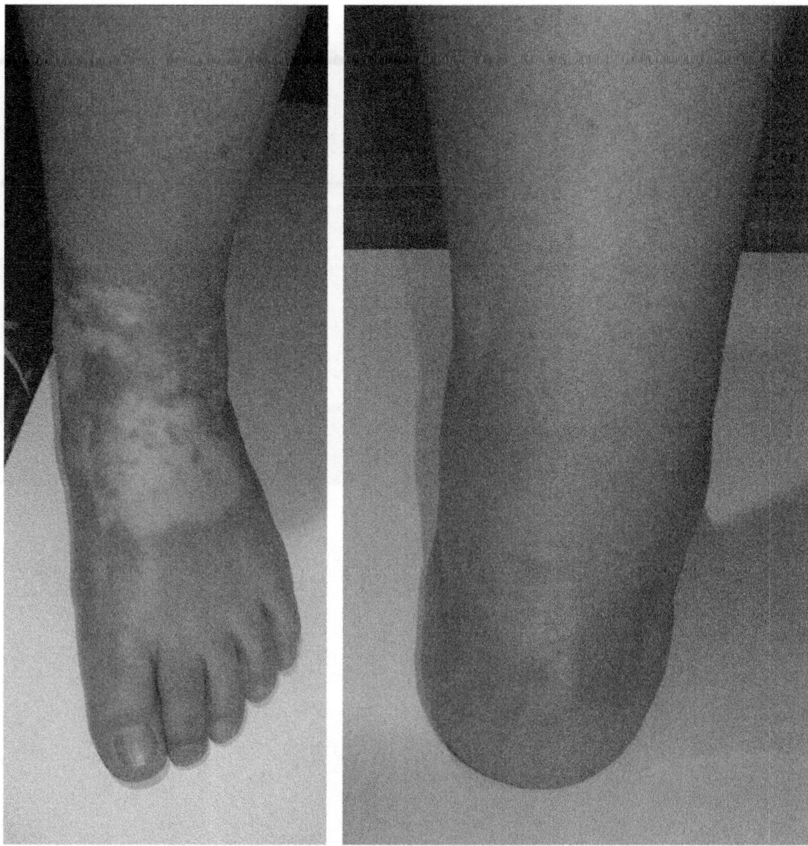

Fig. 5. Final clinical appearance 2 years after the intramedullary nailing of the patient in **Fig. 3**.

loosening of the distal pins from osteopenic disintegrating bone. In addition to the amputation, the complication was drainage from pin holes in 5 and superficial wound infection in one patient. In their study, 5 of 7 (71.4%) of the patients with isolated TT arthrodesis went on to solid union, whereas only 1 of 5 (20.0%) patients requiring TTC fusion obtained a solid union. The remainder of the patients ended with a stable fibrous union that was functional and this was accepted as a success.

Zarutsky and colleagues[38] looked at the use of external fixation for salvage ankle arthrodesis. Of the 43 patients included in the study, 11 patients were treated for CN of the ankle, 5 without additional internal fixation and 6 with internal fixation. All 5 patients without additional internal fixation were able to be salvaged, although one patient required using a wheelchair because of an unstable nonunion. They reported 8 major complications in CN patients. There were 3 (7.3%) below-knee amputations in the whole study group of whom only one was related with CN-associated deep-space infection.

In 2009, Karapinar and colleagues[39] reported 11 patients who had undergone CN ankle reconstruction using Ilizarov external fixators. Of the 11 patients, 10 had successful union at an average of 16.1 weeks and were able to walk freely. The remaining one patient resulted with a fibrous nonunion. At final follow-up, excellent results were obtained in 3 patients, good in 6, fair in 1, and poor in 1.

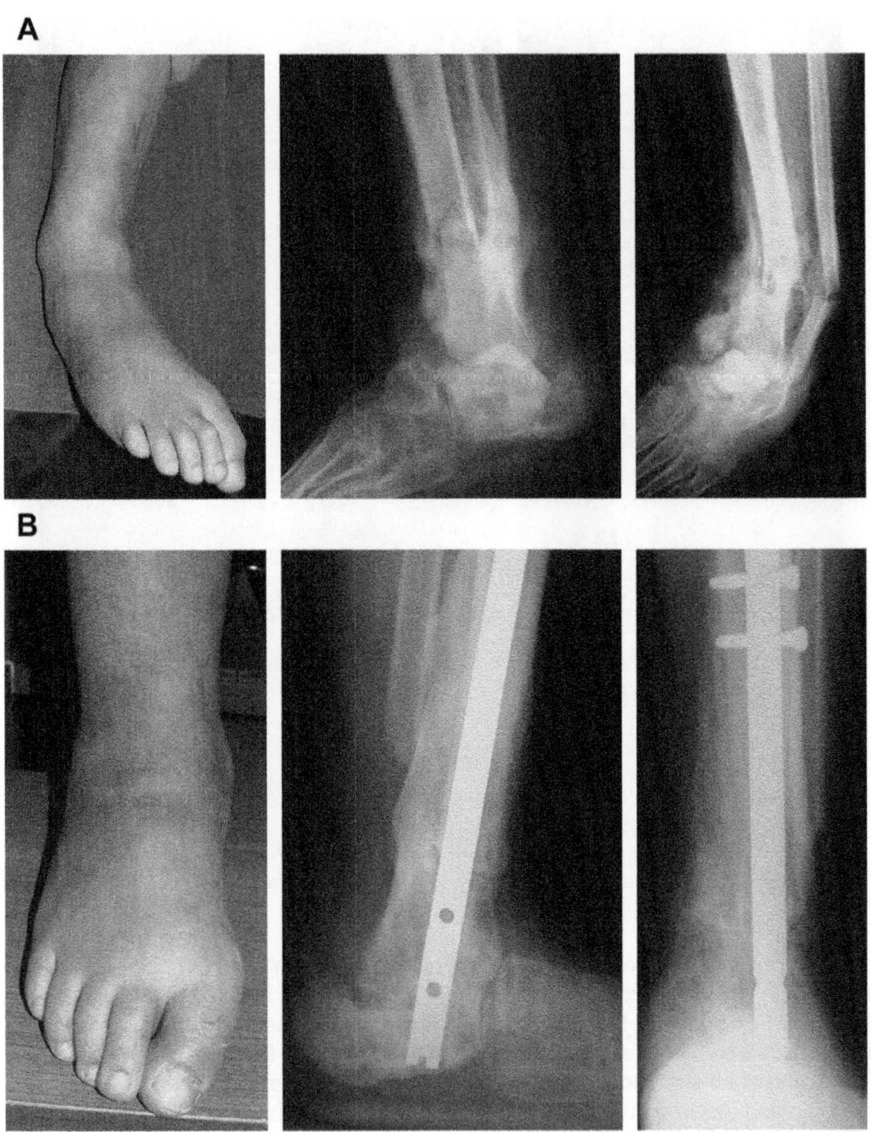

Fig. 6. A 26-year-old patient treated with intramedullary nailing for TTC arthrodesis. Preoperative clinical and radiographic pictures (*A*) followed by clinical and radiographic appearance 4 months after intramedullary nailing (*B*).

In their 2016 study, Ettinger and colleagues[15] used external fixators for ankle CN in 19 of 58 patients. They reported 84.2% fusion rate in external fixator group. In their retrospective study, 2 patients developed deep infectious complications that led to persistent nonunion and ultimately required transtibial amputation.

Condylar Blade Plate

Myerson and colleagues[40] reported the results of internal fixation with adolescent condylar blade plate in 30 patients, 26 of whom had diabetic neuroarthropathy with

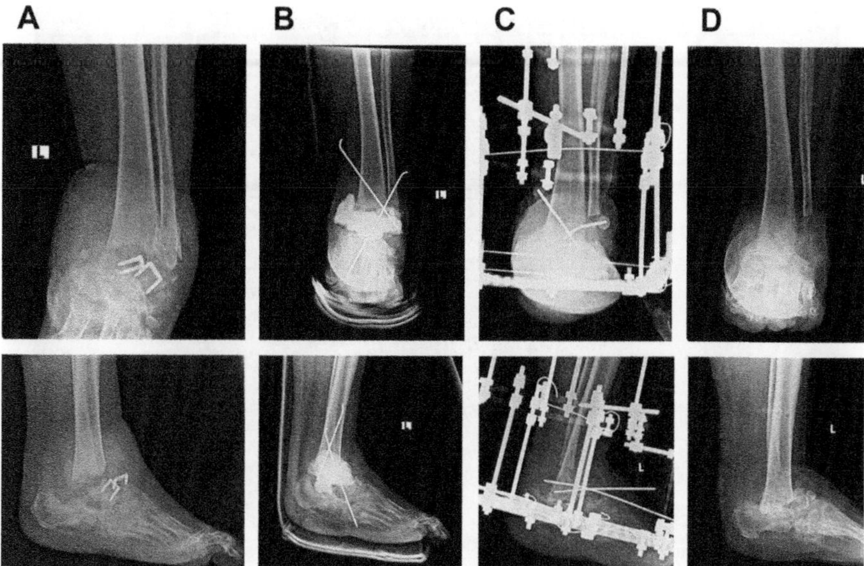

Fig. 7. Anteroposterior and lateral ankle radiographs (*A*) of a 55-year-old woman that presented to the authors' clinic 2 months after she underwent an open reduction and internal fixation with a diagnosis of nondisplaced navicular fracture. Anteroposterior and lateral ankle radiographs after surgical debridement and antibiotic-impregnated cement application (*B*). Anteroposterior and lateral ankle radiographs after further surgical debridement, removal of spacer, and application of external fixation 2 months after the insertion of the antibiotic spacer (*C*). Final anteroposterior and lateral ankle radiographs 4 months after removal of external fixation show fibrous ankylosis (*D*).

talar fragmentation. The surgery was performed with removal of remaining talus, placement of bone graft with antibiotic powder to fill the defect, and fixation with a rigid plate. Fusion was achieved in 28 of 30 patients on average of 16 weeks. There were 2 nonunions, 2 stress fractures at the proximal plate, and 3 superficial infections.

In 2010, Cinar and colleagues[41] reported 100% limb salvage rate in 4 patients with CN of the ankle. They used 95° angled blade plate via a posterior approach for TC arthrodesis and achieved fusion by 5 months in 3 of 4 patients; in the other patient, a stable fibrous ankylosis was achieved (**Fig. 8**).

Locking Plates

Although locking plates are mostly used for the fixation of midfoot CN, they can also be chosen for internal fixation of TC or TTC arthrodesis. Ahmad and colleagues[42] reported 18 cases of TTC fusion using a humeral locking plate, and DiDomenico and Wargo-Dorsey[43] reported on TTC fusion using a femoral locking plate. Similarly, Aikawa and colleagues[44] achieved successful fusion with the use of humeral locking plates for TC arthrodesis in 3 patients. In their study, all patients achieved bony union with a plantigrade foot and without any skin complications.

Combined Fixation

Internal and external fixation can be combined to improve mechanical stability, control adjacent joint mobility, protect the soft tissues, and realign the osseous segments while providing compression and limiting motion to optimize bone healing and

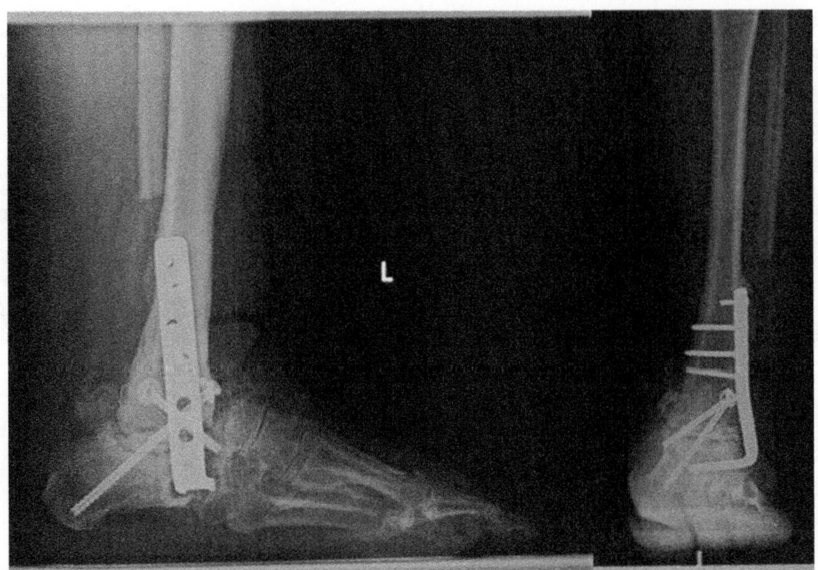

Fig. 8. Lateral and anteroposterior radiographs show an arthrodesis with blade plate and multiple screws.

fusion.[45,46] Hegewald and colleagues[46] combined internal and external fixation in 22 patients with CN. In 6 of 22 patients, TTC arthrodesis were performed for ankle involvement. Two patients (33.33%) in the ankle group developed recurrent deformity, subsequent fixation failure, and required below-knee amputation.

In their series of 52 patients, DeVries and colleagues[30] combined intramedullary nailing with external fixation for 7 patients. There was successful salvage resulting in maintenance of limb in 5 patients (71.4%), and there was no statistically significant difference between the 2 groups in terms of hardware removal, rates of complications, or need for revision surgery.

BONE GRAFTS

Bone grafts can be used to address osseous defects and optimize bone healing in the reconstruction process of diabetic CN-associated deformities. There are several options that can be used. Among these, autogenous bone grafts are the gold standard because of complete histocompatibility and no risk for disease transmission; however, their use is associated with donor-site morbidity, limited supply, and increased surgical time.[47] The most commonly used donor site for autograft harvesting is iliac crest for ankle arthrodesis in CN that is usually harvested from the contralateral hip.[48] Proximal tibia, distal tibia, calcaneus, and fibula can also be used for graft harvesting.[49] The fibula can be used as a strut graft to fill defects and buttress constructs or as an intramedullary graft.[50,51] It can also be prepared as corticocancellous graft to use at the arthrodesis site.

Joint preparation for arthrodesis in CN patients usually leads extensive bone loss, especially in cases with osteomyelitis. Because of the limited supply of autografts, allografts can be used in cases with large bone defects. Femoral head and iliac crest allografts are effective for filling these defects and providing structural support. They can also be used for the restoration of talar height and leg length.[52,53] However, one has to remember that without rigid fixation (which is especially important in cases with CN) abundant use of allograft will not guarantee fusion and can even predispose the surgical site to infection (**Figs. 9** and **10**).

In cases with osteomyelitis, antibiotic-impregnated cement can also be used as a void filler to help soft tissue to heal, to eliminate dead space at the infected bone cavity following surgical debridement, and control infectious process locally without systemic side effects associated with systemic antibiotic use.[54–56]

PRIMARY AMPUTATION

Primary amputation is a choice for some patients, and it may be the most beneficial treatment in certain situations. Patients who are candidates for primary amputation have non-reconstructable peripheral vascular disease, extensive open wound(s) that

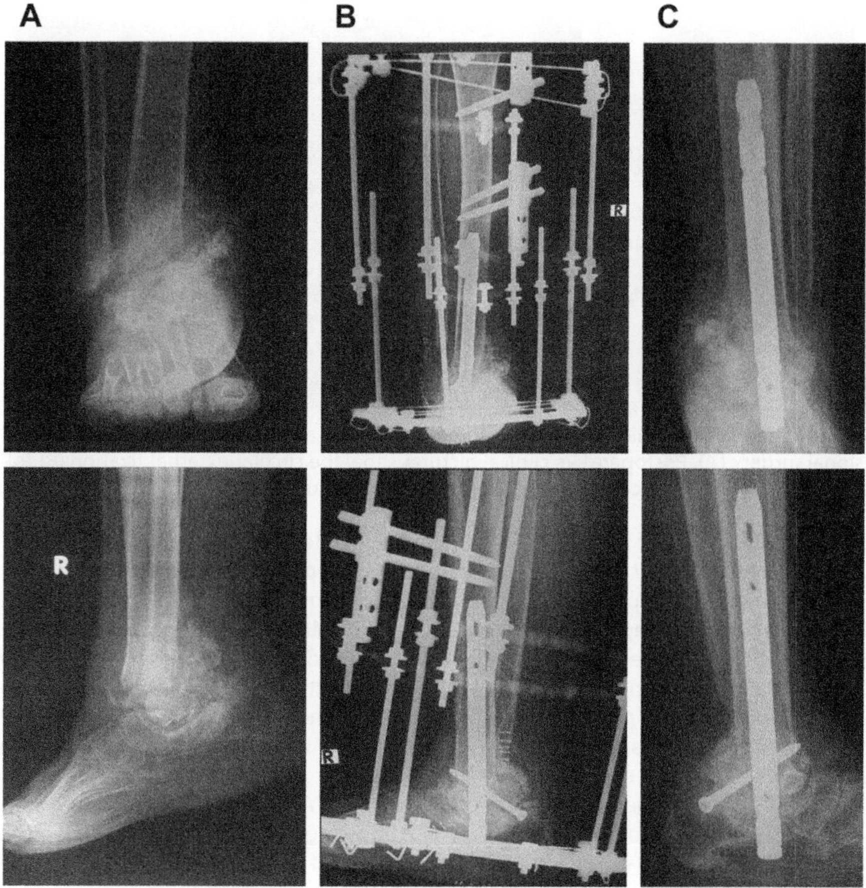

Fig. 9. Preoperative anteroposterior and lateral ankle radiographs (*A*) of an ankle CN that was operated with allograft application and K-wire fixation in another facility (*A*). Five months after her first surgery, the patient presented with pseudoarthrosis, fistulization, and serohemorrhagic drainage. Revisional surgery included combined internal and external fixation and autografting by using the distal fibula (*B*). Final anteroposterior and lateral ankle radiographs 4 months after the revisional surgery (*C*).

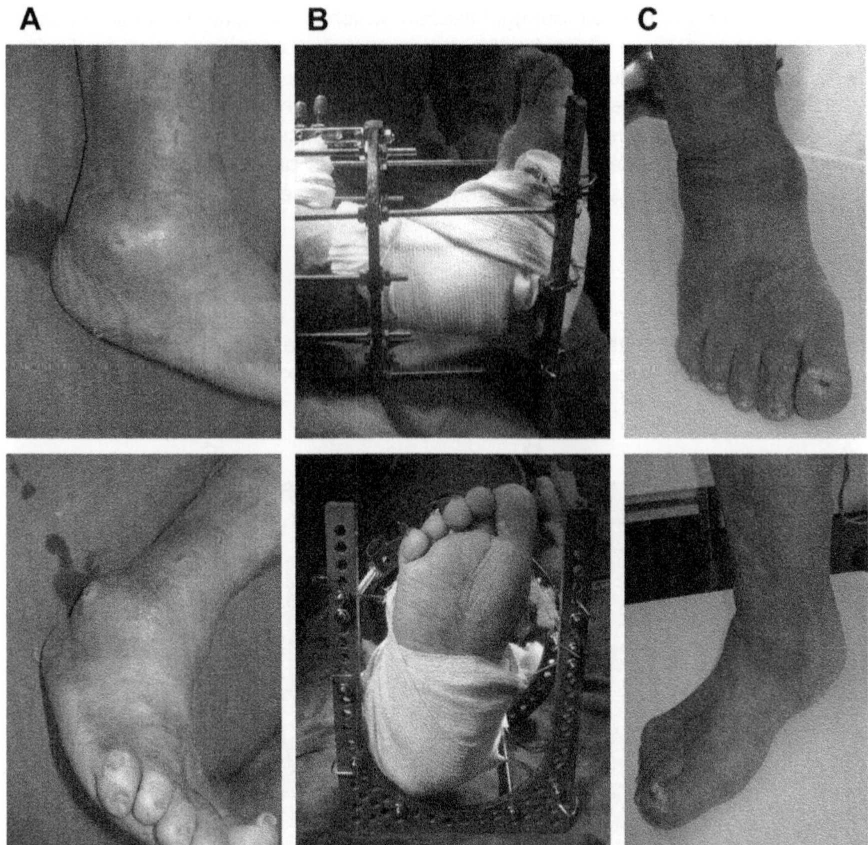

Fig. 10. Preoperative clinical pictures of the same patient as shown in **Fig. 9** before the revisional surgery (*A*). Postoperative clinical pictures show the circular external fixation (*B*) followed by final clinical pictures 4 months after revisional surgery (*C*).

preclude adequate soft tissue coverage, extensive osteomyelitis, multiple comorbidities like renal failure, or a nonambulatory patient and psychiatric disease precluding compliance with the prolonged postoperative regimen.[11] In their recent study, Schneekloth and colleagues[13] reviewed published data regarding the surgical management of CN between 2009 and 2014. They included 30 studies in their review and found an overall amputation rate of 8.9% in patients with CN. Although this number does not reflect the primary amputation rate, it is shown that patients with CN and foot ulcers are 12 times more likely to require a major amputation than patients with CN but without foot ulcers.

Usually below-the-knee amputation is preferred, but Altindas and colleagues[57] suggested a 2-stage Boyd operation technique for late-stage CN feet. All of the patients in their study had hindfoot involvement, and they reported successful results without any complications, with a mean follow-up of 2.1 years with their technique.

SUMMARY

CN is associated with progressive, noninfectious, osteolysis-induced bone and joint destruction. When ankle and/or hindfoot is affected by the destruction process, the clinical presentation is further complicated with collapse and destruction of the talar body, which increases instability around the ankle. In this patient population, arthrodesis is the most commonly used surgical procedure. Internal fixation, external fixation, or a combination of both can be used for the surgical reconstruction. Decision making between them should be individualized according to the patient characteristics.

REFERENCES

1. Güven MF, Karabiber A, Kaynak G, et al. Conservative and surgical treatment of the chronic Charcot foot and ankle. Diabet Foot Ankle 2013;4.
2. Sanders LJ, Fryberg RG. The Charcot foot. In: Bowker JH, Pfeifer MA, editors. Levin and O'Neal's the diabetic foot. 7th edition. Philadelphia: Mosby Elsevier; 2007. p. 257–83.
3. Miller DS, Lichtman WF. Diabetic neuropathic arthropathy of feet; summary report of seventeen cases. AMA Arch Surg 1955;70:513–8.
4. La Fontaine J, Lavery L, Jude E. Current concepts of Charcot foot in diabetic patients. Foot (Edinb) 2015;26:7–14.
5. Eichenholtz S. Charcot joints. Springfield (IL): Charles C Thomas; 1966.
6. Brodsky JW, Rouse AM. Exostectomy for symptomatic bony prominences in diabetic Charcot feet. Clin Orthop Relat Res 1993;296:21–6.
7. Sanders LJ, Frykberg RG. Diabetic neuropathic osteoarthropathy. the Charcot foot. In: Frykberg RG, editor. The high risk foot in diabetes mellitus. New York: Churchill Livingston; 1991. p. 297.
8. Schon LC, Weinfeld SB, Horton GA, et al. Radiographic and clinical classification of acquired midtarsus deformities. Foot Ankle Int 1998;19:394–404.
9. Scott RT, DeCarbo WT, Hyer CF. Osteotomies for the management of charcot neuroarthropathy of the foot and ankle. Clin Podiatr Med Surg 2015;32:405–18.
10. Varma AK. Charcot neuroarthropathy of the foot and ankle: a review. J Foot Ankle Surg 2013;52:740–9.
11. Johnson JE, Klein SE, Brodsky JW. Diabetes. In: Coughlin MJ, Saltzman CL, Anderson RB, editors. Mann's surgery of the foot and ankle. Philadelphia: Mosby Elsevier; 2014. p. 1385–480.
12. Robinson AH, Pasapula C, Brodsky JW. Surgical aspects of the diabetic foot. J Bone Joint Surg Br 2009;91:1–7.
13. Schneekloth BJ, Lowery NJ, Wukich DK. Charcot neuroarthropathy in patients with diabetes: an updated systematic review of surgical management. J Foot Ankle Surg 2016;55(3):586–90.
14. Burns PR, Wukich DK. Surgical reconstruction of the Charcot rearfoot and ankle. Clin Podiatr Med Surg 2008;25:95–120.
15. Ettinger S, Plaass C, Claassen L, et al. Surgical management of Charcot deformity for the foot and ankle-radiologic outcome after internal/external fixation. J Foot Ankle Surg 2016;55(3):522–8.
16. Stapleton JJ, Belczyk R, Zgonis T. Revisional Charcot foot and ankle surgery. Clin Podiatr Med Surg 2009;26:127–39.
17. Garapati R, Weinfeld SB. Complex reconstruction of the diabetic foot and ankle. Am J Surg 2004;187:81S–6S.
18. Lowery NJ, Woods JB, Armstrong DG, et al. Surgical management of Charcot neuroarthropathy of the foot and ankle: a systematic review. Foot Ankle Int 2012;33:113–21.
19. Kim JY, Hwang S, Lee Y. Selective plantar fascia release for nonhealing diabetic plantar ulcerations. J Bone Joint Surg Am 2012;94:1297–302.

20. Holstein P, Lohmann M, Bitsch M, et al. Achilles tendon lengthening, the panacea for plantar forefoot ulceration? Diabetes Metab Res Rev 2004;20:S37–40.
21. Shen W, Wukich D. Orthopaedic surgery and the diabetic Charcot foot. Med Clin North Am 2013;97:873–82.
22. Wukich DK, Raspovic KM, Hobizal KB, et al. Surgical management of Charcot neuroarthropathy of the ankle and hindfoot in patients with diabetes. Diabetes Metab Res Rev 2016;32:292–6.
23. Siebachmeyer M, Boddu K, Bilal A, et al. Outcome of one-stage correction of deformities of the ankle and hindfoot and fusion in Charcot neuroarthropathy using a retrograde intramedullary hindfoot arthrodesis nail. Bone Joint J 2015;97:76–82.
24. Cooper PS. Application of external fixators for management of Charcot deformities of the foot and ankle. Foot Ankle Clin 2002;7:207–54.
25. Pinzur MS. The role of ring external fixation in Charcot foot arthropathy. Foot Ankle Clin 2006;11:837–47.
26. Herbst SA. External fixation of Charcot arthropathy. Foot Ankle Clin 2004;9:595–609.
27. Jolly GP, Zgonis T, Polyzois V. External fixation in the management of Charcot neuroarthropathy. Clin Podiatr Med Surg 2003;20:741–56.
28. Tisdel CL, Marcus RE, Heiple KG. Triple arthrodesis for diabetic peritalar neuroarthropathy. Foot Ankle Int 1995;16:332–8.
29. Early JS, Hansen ST. Surgical reconstruction of the diabetic foot: a salvage approach for midfoot collapse. Foot Ankle Int 1996;17:325–30.
30. DeVries JG, Berlet GC, Hyer CF. A retrospective comparative analysis of Charcot ankle stabilization using an intramedullary rod with or without application of circular external fixator–utilization of the Retrograde Arthrodesis Intramedullary Nail database. J Foot Ankle Surg 2012;51:420–5.
31. Dayton P, Feilmeier M, Thompson M, et al. Comparison of complications for internal and external fixation for charcot reconstruction: a systematic review. J Foot Ankle Surg 2015;54:1072–5.
32. Caravaggi C, Cimmino M, Caruso S, et al. Intramedullary compressive nail fixation for the treatment of severe Charcot deformity of the ankle and rear foot. J Foot Ankle Surg 2006;45:20–4.
33. Dalla Paola L, Volpe A, Varotto D, et al. Use of a retrograde nail for ankle arthrodesis in Charcot neuroarthropathy: a limb salvage procedure. Foot Ankle Int 2007;28:967–70.
34. Farber DC, Juliano PJ, Cavanagh PR, et al. Single stage correction with external fixation of the ulcerated foot in individuals with Charcot neuroarthropathy. Foot Ankle Int 2002;23:130–4.
35. Pinzur MS. Current concepts review: Charcot arthropathy of the foot and ankle. Foot Ankle Int 2007;28:952–9.
36. Ogut T, Glisson RR, Chuckpaiwong B, et al. External ring fixation versus screw fixation for ankle arthrodesis: a biomechanical comparison. Foot Ankle Int 2009;30:353–60.
37. Fabrin J, Larsen K, Holstein PE. Arthrodesis with external fixation in the unstable of misaligned Charcot ankle in patients with diabetes mellitus. Int J Low Extrem Wounds 2007;6:102–7.
38. Zarutsky E, Rush SM, Schuberth JM. The use of circular wire external fixation in the treatment of salvage ankle arthrodesis. J Foot Ankle Surg 2005;44:22–31.
39. Karapinar H, Sener M, Kazimoglu C, et al. Arthrodesis of neuropathic ankle joint by Ilizarov fixator in diabetic patients. J Am Podiatr Med Assoc 2009;99:42–8.

40. Myerson MS, Alvarez RG, Lam PW. Tibiocalcaneal arthrodesis for the management of severe ankle and hindfoot deformities. Foot Ankle Int 2000;21:643–50.
41. Cinar M, Derincek A, Akpinar S. Tibiocalcaneal arthrodesis with posterior blade plate in diabetic neuroarthropthy. Foot Ankle Int 2010;31:511–6.
42. Ahmad J, Pour AE, Raikin SM. The modified use of a proximal humeral locking plate for tibiotalocalcaneal arthrodesis. Foot Ankle Int 2007;28:977–83.
43. DiDomenico LA, Wargo-Dorsey M. Tibiotalocalcaneal arthrodesis using a femoral locking plate. J Foot Ankle Surg 2012;51:128–32.
44. Aikawa T, Watanabe K, Matsubara H, et al. Tibiocalcaneal fusion for Charcot ankle with severe talar body loss: case report and a review of the surgical literature. J Foot Ankle Surg 2016;55:247–51.
45. Stapleton JJ, Zgonis T. Surgical reconstruction of the diabetic Charcot foot: internal, external or combined fixation? Clin Podiatr Med Surg 2012;29:425–33.
46. Hegewald KW, Wilder ML, Chappell TM, et al. Combined internal and external fixation for diabetic Charcot reconstruction: a retrospective case series. J Foot Ankle Surg 2016;55(3):619–27.
47. Fitzgibbons TC, Hawks MA, McMullen ST, et al. Bone grafting in surgery about the foot and ankle: indications and techniques. J Am Acad Orthop Surg 2011; 19:112–20.
48. Zgonis T, Stapleton JJ, Jeffries LC, et al. Surgical treatment of Charcot neuropathy. AORN J 2008;87:971–86.
49. Ramanujam CL, Facaros Z, Zgonis T. An overview of bone grafting techniques for the diabetic Charcot foot and ankle. Clin Podiatr Med Surg 2012;29:589–95.
50. Jeong ST, Park HB, Hwang SC, et al. Use of intramedullary nonvascularized fibular graft with external fixation for revisional Charcot ankle fusion: a case report. J Foot Ankle Surg 2012;51:249–53.
51. Paul J, Barg A, Horisberger M, et al. Ankle salvage surgery with autologous circular pillar fibula augmentation and intramedullary hindfoot nail. J Foot Ankle Surg 2014;53:601–5.
52. Thomason K, Eyres KS. A technique of fusion for failed total replacement of the ankle: tibio-allograft-calcaneal fusion with a locked retrograde intramedullary nail. J Bone Joint Surg Br 2008;90:885–8.
53. Jeng CL, Campbell JT, Tang EY, et al. Tibiotalocalcaneal arthrodesis with bulk femoral head allograft for salvage of large defects in the ankle. Foot Ankle Int 2013;34:1256–66.
54. Hong CC, Jin Tan K, Lahiri A, et al. Use of a definitive cement spacer for simultaneous bony and soft tissue reconstruction of mid- and hindfoot diabetic neuroarthropathy: a case report. J Foot Ankle Surg 2015;54:120–5.
55. Stapleton JJ, Zgonis T. Concomitant osteomyelitis and avascular necrosis of the talus treated with talectomy and tibiocalcaneal arthrodesis. Clin Podiatr Med Surg 2013;30:251–6.
56. Ramanujam CL, Zgonis T. Antibiotic-loaded cement beads for Charcot ankle osteomyelitis. Foot Ankle Spec 2010;3:274–7.
57. Altindas M, Kilic A, Ceber M. A new limb-salvaging technique for the treatment of late stage complicated Charcot foot deformity: two-staged Boyd's operation. Foot Ankle Surg 2012;18:190–4.

Soft Tissue Reconstruction Pyramid for the Diabetic Charcot Foot

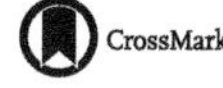

Claire M. Capobianco, DPM[a,*], Thomas Zgonis, DPM[b]

KEYWORDS

• Diabetic foot ulcer • Diabetic Charcot foot • Charcot neuroarthropathy
• Soft tissue pyramid • Diabetic neuropathy • Plastic surgery • Reconstruction

KEY POINTS

- Durable soft tissue coverage is essential for the surgical treatment of soft tissue and/or osseous defects in the diabetic Charcot neuroarthropathy (DCN) patient.
- The soft tissue reconstruction pyramid for the DCN patient provides a stepwise approach when managing challenging acute or chronic soft tissue defects.
- Concomitant osteomyelitis in DCN ulcers is optimally addressed with combined osseous and vascularized soft tissue transfer reconstruction.
- External fixation may be used as an adjunctive therapy for surgical off-loading of major soft tissue reconstruction for DCN ulcers.

The incidence of foot ulceration in the diabetic population has been cited as 15%,[1] and in the diabetic Charcot neuroarthropathy (DCN) population, the incidence climbs to 37%.[2] The evidence of the financial burden of diabetic foot ulceration (DFU) treatment[3–11] as well as the negative effect on patient quality of life associated with chronic DFU is staggering.[5,12] In addition, DFU recurrence rates of 25% to 80% have been published, despite enrollment in diabetic shoe programs and regular podiatric visits.[13–16] In addition, the mortality risk of patients with DFU or DCN has been shown to be higher than that for patients with diabetes mellitus alone.[17] The data in this high-risk diabetic population underscore the importance of a durable and reproducible surgical treatment approach to these difficult DCN ulcers when conservative therapy fails.

Disclosure: The authors have nothing to disclose. T. Zgonis is the Consulting Editor for the *Clinics in Podiatric Medicine and Surgery.*

[a] Orthopaedic Associates of Southern Delaware, 1539 Savannah Road, Suite 203, Lewes, DE 19958, USA; [b] Division of Podiatric Medicine and Surgery, Department of Orthopaedics, University of Texas Health Science Center San Antonio, 7703 Floyd Curl Drive, MSC 7776, San Antonio, TX 78229, USA
* Corresponding author.
E-mail address: ccapobianco@delawarebonedocs.com

Clin Podiatr Med Surg 34 (2017) 69–76
http://dx.doi.org/10.1016/j.cpm.2016.07.008 podiatric.theclinics.com

Patients with DCN carry the heavy burden of multiple end-organ manifestations of the primary disease. In addition, these patients often have multiple other medical comorbidities, including microvascular and macrovascular peripheral arterial disease, cardiac disease, end-stage renal disease, retinopathy, gastroparesis, and autonomic neuropathy. Preoperative medical optimization of these patients often requires a multidisciplinary team approach and may involve the patient's primary care physician, cardiologist, endocrinologist, nutritionist, nephrologist, infectious disease specialist, and/or vascular surgeon. A thorough history, physical examination, and preoperative laboratory and medical imaging are paramount for the patient's overall successful outcome.

In the presence of DCN and concomitant osteomyelitis or abscess, staged reconstruction is necessary before the final soft tissue coverage and/or osseous reconstruction. Initial multiple surgical debridements, osseous resections, and/or utilization of cemented non-biodegradable antibiotic beads/spacers may be required in order to achieve healthy wound and osseous margins before the definitive surgical reconstruction. Furthermore, basic arterial noninvasive studies are highly recommended in diabetic patients with diminished pulses or signs of peripheral arterial insufficiency. Vascular surgery consultation is warranted in the presence of diminished ankle brachial index, large vessel obstructive disease, or monophasic blunted waveforms to the feet.[18]

The options for soft tissue coverage in the patient with DCN are usually based on anatomic location, size and depth of the ulceration, durability of surrounding soft tissue, the presence or absence of active infection, and underlying deformity. Soft tissue coverage options are often affected by the patient's specific angiology. The reconstructive ladder is a classic tenet of plastic surgery in which tissue coverage techniques are arranged hierarchically from simple to complex. The techniques are applied accordingly based on the soft tissue defect characteristics and were revised recently specifically for patients with diabetes mellitus.[19] In patients with DCN, the ulcerations are more complicated with or without the presence of osteomyelitis and are usually associated with an underlying deformity. As a result, the bottom rungs of the reconstructive soft tissue pyramid[19] (skin equivalents, negative pressure wound therapy, or autogenous skin grafting) are generally used less frequently, owing to the complexities of DCN ulcerations. Ulcer excision with or without exostectomy and/or equinus correction and primary closure of DCN ulcers is the simplest method of soft tissue coverage, but this is often not possible secondary to the size of the wound or the lack of redundant and durable surrounding soft tissue.

SOFT TISSUE COVERAGE OPTIONS FOR THE DIABETIC CHARCOT FOOT

Local Random Flaps

Local random flaps make up the next step in the soft tissue reconstructive pyramid for DCN ulcers (**Fig. 1**). These flaps include the skin, subcutaneous tissue, and sometimes the fascia. The flaps are random in nature without any specific arterial blood supply and may be sometimes based on angiosomes. Bilobed variants[20] and V-Y random advancement flaps may be used for coverage of plantar or malleolar defects, as long as no underlying osteomyelitis is present.[21–24]

Most common local random flaps for soft tissue coverage of DCN ulcerations include the rotational advancement, transpositional, rhomboid, and/or monolobe/bilobed flaps. The use of local rotational advancement flaps based on the medial plantar arterial angiosome is frequently used for plantar-lateral midfoot ulcers in the DCN patient.[25–27] Noninvasive arterial studies are crucial for preoperative planning

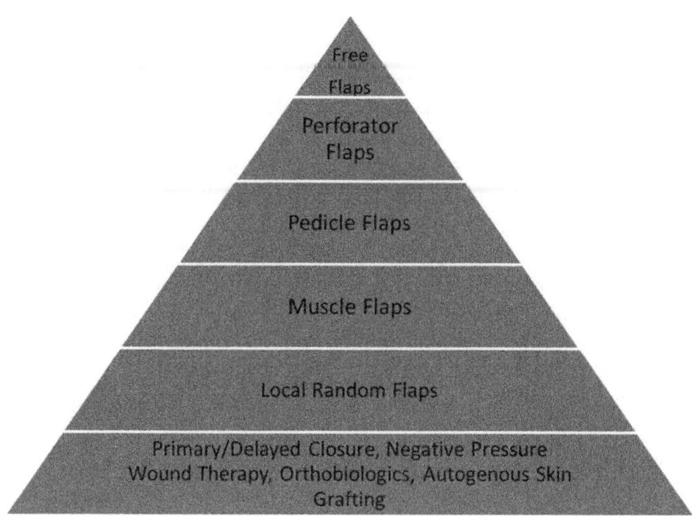

Fig. 1. The soft tissue reconstructive pyramid for surgical reconstruction of the diabetic Charcot foot.

as weak posterior tibial artery inflow precludes the successful application of this flap. In some cases, the plantar fascia is often incorporated into this designed flap for additional durability.[28] The non-weight-bearing donor site is typically covered with an autogenous split-thickness skin graft or skin-equivalent bioengineered tissue graft. Surgical off-loading with circular external fixation may also be indicated in certain clinical case scenarios where the underlying deformity and equinus are simultaneously addressed at the time of surgical reconstruction.

Local Muscle Flaps

Local muscle flaps constitute the next step in the soft tissue reconstructive pyramid for DCN ulcers.[29,30] The flexor digitorum brevis, abductor hallucis, abductor digiti minimi, and extensor digitorum brevis muscle flaps have all been described for the DCN patient.[30] Local muscle flaps are most appropriate when wide osseous or joint resections are performed in cases of osteomyelitis or when the soft tissue defect is in a weight-bearing portion of the foot. Soft tissue coverage with a local muscle flap provides a highly vascularized tissue bed, which is advantageous for healing and long-term durability. In DCN, muscle flaps offer excellent local perfusion to the surgical site following resection of contiguous osteomyelitis of the cuboid or cuneiforms[31]; the increased local perfusion aids in surgical site healing and in delivery of concomitant parenteral antibiotic therapy. Preoperative vascular arterial testing is also crucial for planning of the appropriate local muscle flap design. Muscle flaps can be harvested alone and covered with autogenous skin graft or allograft, or may be transferred en bloc with the overlying skin as musculocutaneous flaps.

The flexor digitorum brevis muscle flap is a durable option for plantar central ulcerations resulting from DCN collapse. The success of this flap as an option is predicated on sufficient size of the muscle belly and absence of prior muscular debulking from infection or surgical debridement. MRI may aid in preoperative planning if the integrity of the flexor digitorum brevis muscle is uncertain.[29] This flap is supplied by muscular branches of the lateral and medial plantar arteries and associated metatarsal/digital arteries, which are meticulously preserved intraoperatively. The associated tendons from the plantar aspects of the second, third, and/or fourth toes are transected distally and used to help mobilize, dissect, and rotate the flap proximally.

The abductor hallucis muscle flap may be useful for soft tissue coverage in DCN plantar medial ulcers, metatarsal head defects, plantar central defects, and with sufficient bulk and dissection, for medial malleolar defects.[29–31] This flap is also supplied by muscular branches of the medial plantar artery, which are readily identifiable with careful dissection. The abductor digiti minimi muscle flap may be applied to DCN plantar lateral ulcers and lateral calcaneal ulcerations and is supplied by muscular branches of the lateral plantar artery.[29] The extensor digitorum brevis muscle flap may be used for dorsolateral proximal wounds caused by DCN collapse and/or osteomyelitis. This flap is mainly supplied by the muscular branches of the dorsalis pedis artery. Muscle flaps require the concomitant application of autogenous split thickness skin grafts or skin-equivalent bioengineered grafts when harvested alone. A bolster dressing or negative pressure dressing is used to secure the harvested muscle flap-skin graft construct to reduce shear force and prevent any underlying hematoma formation.

Local and Distant Pedicle Flaps

Local or distant pedicle flaps are harvested with the associated neurovascular supply and may be designed with retrograde or anterograde vascular infow.[32] Pedicle flaps may be indicated when other reconstructive efforts have failed, or if the soft tissue defect size or location is not amenable to other soft tissue coverage options. An intimate understanding of the angiosomes in the foot and ankle as well as vascular assessment and intervention when necessary is a prerequisite for preoperative planning.[33] The most common local pedicle flap used in the DCN reconstruction is the medial plantar artery flap.

The medial plantar artery flap is usually used to cover large plantar forefoot, midfoot, or heel soft tissue defects.[32,34,35] Preoperative Doppler ultrasound is used to map the medial plantar artery before surgery. If greater mobility is needed, the medial plantar artery flap may be designed as an island flap, with the superficial branch of the medial plantar artery supplying the entire flap. Alternatively, if a medial skin bridge is maintained, the perforating deep plantar branch of the dorsalis pedis artery provides collateral inflow to the flap.[36,37] The lateral plantar artery flap may also be used for large weight-bearing areas of the DCN.[38] For hindfoot/ankle DCN ulcers, the reverse flow sural neurofasciocutaneous pedicle flap is used to cover large soft tissue defects with or without associated arthrodesis procedures.[39]

Perforator and Free Flaps

The use of perforator flaps usually based on the peroneal artery may be useful in the diabetic lower extremity reconstruction or in the DCN patient with concomitant osteomyelitis of the hindfoot/ankle. These flaps are dependent on a patent peroneal artery, which is identified by preoperative vascular medical imaging.[40–42] The donor leg sites are usually covered with an autogenous split-thickness skin graft or skin graft substitute. Surgical off-loading with external fixation may also be necessary when simultaneous osseous correction is performed in the DCN patient. Free tissue transfer for soft tissue coverage of DCN ulcers is rarely used in the diabetic patient with multiple medical comorbidities. Some of the major concerns of free tissue transfers include and are not limited to increased recipient and donor site complications, extensive surgical duration and anesthesia exposure, vascular anastomosic concerns in the

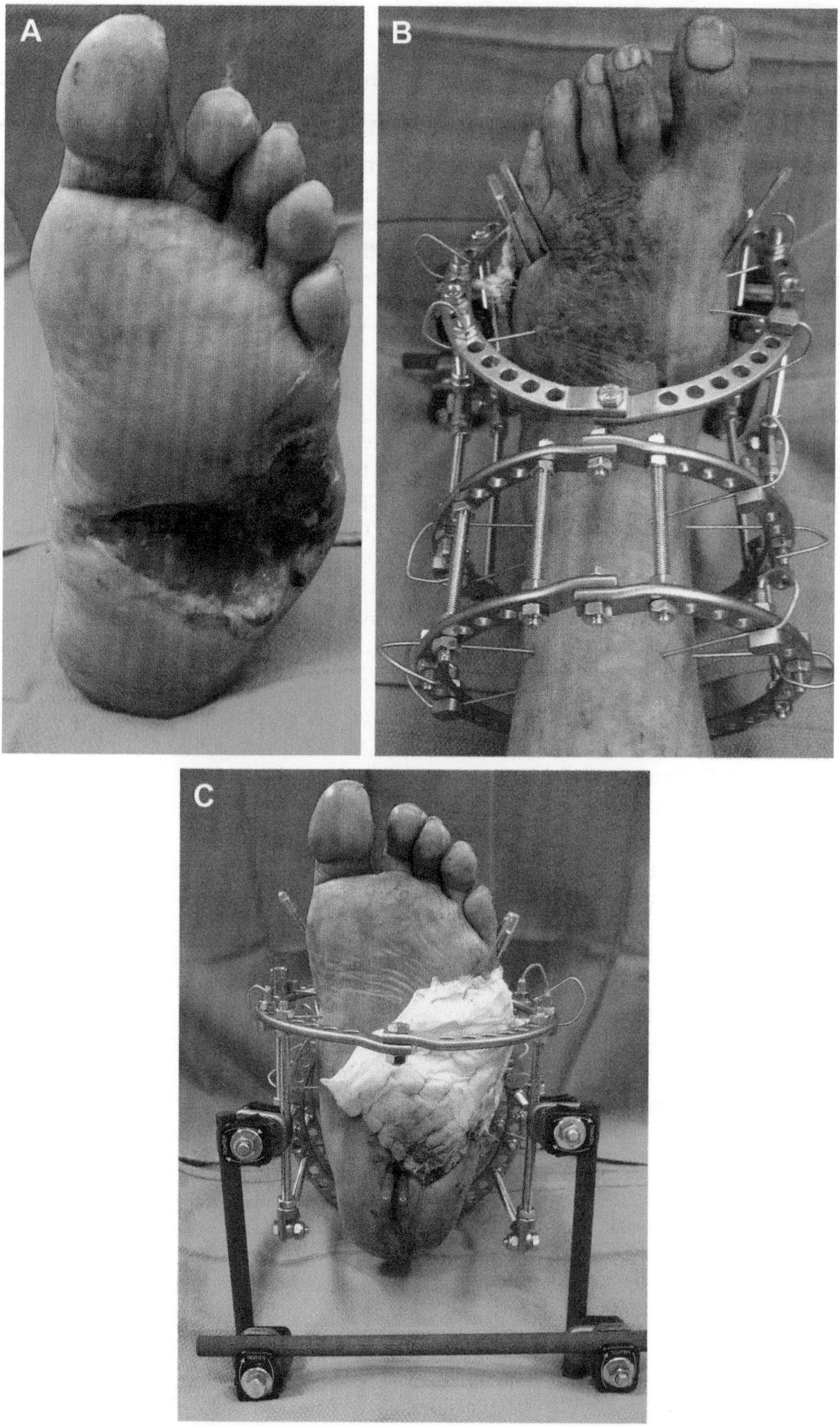

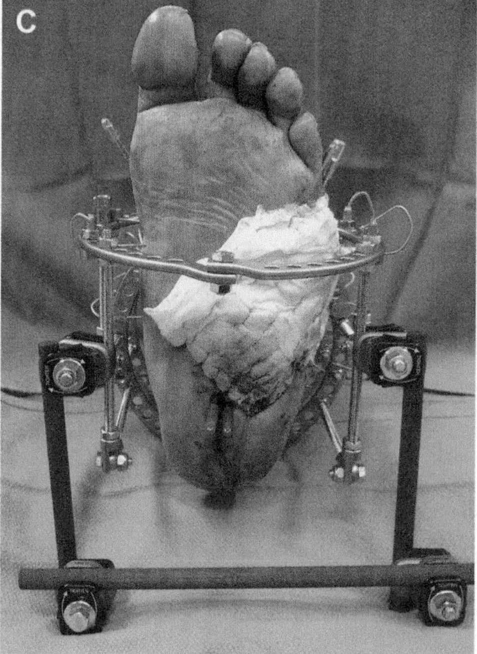

Fig. 2. Intraoperative clinical picture shows a severe soft tissue and osseous defect in a patient with diabetic Charcot neuroathropathy (*A*) that required staged reconstructions, including lateral column arthrodesis, allografting, foot and ankle stabilization, and circular external fixation (*B, C*).

presence of diabetic arterial calcifications, and diseased or absent pedal target vessels.[43,44]

In addition, adjunctive external fixation may also be a useful tool for any type of soft tissue reconstructive procedure on the weight-bearing surface of the DCN patient.[45] External fixation facilitates soft tissue quiescence by preventing motion and limiting shear and weight-bearing stresses to the foot and ankle. In the diabetic neuropathic population, external fixation can successfully prevent inappropriate weight-bearing on fragile soft tissue reconstructions (**Fig. 2**).[24–27,45–47]

SUMMARY

Soft tissue coverage in the DCN patient can be complicated secondary to degree of osseous deformity, medical comorbidities, and the ramifications of the underlying end-organ disease state. Diligent preoperative planning and a multidisciplinary approach are advised for optimal outcomes. A hierarchy of available options for soft tissue reconstruction in the DCN patient is applied based on the history, location, size, chronicity, infection, and complexity of the defect with great emphasis on the patient's individual anatomy. The soft tissue reconstructive pyramid described for the DCN patient offers the reconstructive surgeon a logical anatomic approach to managing challenging soft tissue and/or osseous defects.

REFERENCES

1. Andros G, Armstrong DG, Attinger CE, et al. Consensus statement on negative pressure wound therapy (V.A.C. Therapy) for the management of diabetic foot wounds. Ostomy Wound Manage 2006;(Suppl):1–32.
2. Larsen K, Fabrin J, Holstein PE. Incidence and management of ulcers in diabetic Charcot feet. J Wound Care 2001;10:323–8.
3. Centers for Disease Control and Prevention. National Diabetes Fact Sheet 2007. Available at: www.cdc.gov/diabetes/pubs/factsheet07.htm. Accessed March 6, 2010.
4. Apelqvist J, Armstrong DG, Lavery LA, et al. Resource utilization and economic costs of care based on a randomized trial of vacuum-assisted closure therapy in the treatment of diabetic foot wounds. Am J Surg 2008;195:782–8.
5. Rerkasem K, Kosachunhanun N, Tongprasert S, et al. A multidisciplinary diabetic foot protocol at Chiang Mai University Hospital: cost and quality of life. Int J Low Extrem Wounds 2009;8:153–6.
6. Siriwardana HD, Weerasekera D. The cost of diabetic foot conditions. Ceylon Med J 2007;52:89–91.
7. Redekop WK, Stolk EA, Kok E, et al. Diabetic foot ulcers and amputations: estimates of health utility for use in cost-effectiveness analyses of new treatments. Diabetes Metab 2004;30:549–56.
8. Girod I, Valensi P, Laforet C, et al. An economic evaluation of the cost of diabetic foot ulcers: results of a retrospective study on 239 patients. Diabetes Metab 2003;29:269–77.
9. Ortegon MM, Redekop WK, Niessen LW. Cost-effectiveness of prevention and treatment of the diabetic foot: a Markov analysis. Diabetes Care 2004;27:901–7.
10. Albert S. Cost-effective management of recalcitrant diabetic foot ulcers. Clin Podiatr Med Surg 2002;19:483–91.
11. Kantor J, Margolis DJ. Treatment options for diabetic neuropathic foot ulcers: a cost-effectiveness analysis. Dermatol Surg 2001;27:347–51.

12. Roukis TS, Stapleton JJ, Zgonis T. Addressing psychosocial aspects of care for patients with diabetes undergoing limb salvage surgery. Clin Podiatr Med Surg 2007;24:601–10.
13. Uccioli L, Faglia E, Monticone G, et al. Manufactured shoes in the prevention of diabetic foot ulcers. Diabetes Care 1995;18:1376–8.
14. Mueller MJ, Sinacore DR, Hastings MK, et al. Effect of Achilles tendon lengthening on neuropathic plantar ulcers: a randomized clinical trial. J Bone Joint Surg Am 2003;85:1436–45.
15. Chantelau E, Kushner T, Spraul M. How effective is cushioned therapeutic footwear in protecting diabetic feet? A clinical study. Diabet Med 1990;7:355–9.
16. Busch K, Chantelau E. Effectiveness of a new brand of stock 'diabetic' shoes to protect against diabetic foot ulcer relapse. A prospective cohort study. Diabet Med 2003;20:665–9.
17. Sohn MW, Lee TA, Stuck RM, et al. Mortality risk of Charcot arthropathy compared with that of diabetic foot ulcer and diabetes alone. Diabetes Care 2009;32: 816–21.
18. Aust MC, Spies M, Guggenheim M, et al. Lower limb revascularisation preceding surgical wound coverage—an interdisciplinary algorithm for chronic wound closure. J Plast Reconstr Aesthet Surg 2008;61:925–33.
19. Capobianco CM, Stapleton JJ, Zgonis T. Soft tissue reconstruction pyramid in the diabetic foot. Foot Ankle Spec 2010;3:241–8.
20. Yetkin H, Kanatli U, Ozturk AM, et al. Bilobed flaps for nonhealing ulcer treatment. Foot Ankle Int 2003;24:685–9.
21. Giraldo F, De Haro F, Ferrer A. Opposed transverse extended V-Y plantar flaps for reconstruction of neuropathic metatarsal head ulcers. Plast Reconstr Surg 2001; 108:1019–24.
22. Eroglu L, Guneren E, Keskin M, et al. The extended V-Y flap for coverage of a mid-planatar defect. Br J Plast Surg 2000;53:708–10.
23. Capobianco CM, Ramanujam CL, Zgonis T. A simple adjunct to a plantar local random flap for submetatarsal ulcers. Clin Podiatr Med Surg 2010;27:167–72.
24. Belczyk R, Stapleton JJ, Zgonis T. A case report of a double advancement flap closure combined with an Ilizarov technique for the chronic plantar forefoot ulceration. Int J Low Extrem Wounds 2009;8:31–6.
25. Zgonis T, Stapleton JJ, Roukis TS. Advanced plastic surgery techniques for soft tissue coverage of the diabetic foot. Clin Podiatr Med Surg 2007;24:547–68.
26. Stapleton JJ, Belczyk R, Zgonis T. Revisional Charcot foot and ankle surgery. Clin Podiatr Med Surg 2009;26:127–39.
27. Zgonis T, Roukis TS, Stapleton JJ, et al. Combined lateral column arthrodesis, medial plantar artery flap, and circular external fixation for Charcot midfoot collapse with chronic plantar ulceration. Adv Skin Wound Care 2008;21:521–5.
28. Altindas M, Cinar C. Promoting primary healing after ray amputations in the diabetic foot: the plantar dermo-fat pad flap. Plast Reconstr Surg 2005;116:1029–34.
29. Attinger CE, Ducic I, Cooper P, et al. The role of intrinsic muscle flaps of the foot for bone coverage in foot and ankle defects in diabetic and nondiabetic patients. Plast Reconstr Surg 2002;110:1047–54.
30. Ramanujam CL, Zgonis T. Versatility of intrinsic muscle flaps for the diabetic Charcot foot. Clin Podiatr Med Surg 2012;29:323–6.
31. Capobianco CM, Zgonis T. Abductor hallucis muscle flap and staged medial column arthrodesis for the chronic ulcerated Charcot foot with concomitant osteomyelitis. Foot Ankle Spec 2010;3:269–73.

32. Pallua N, Di Benedetto G, Berger A. Forefoot reconstruction by reversed island flaps in diabetic patients. Plast Reconstr Surg 2000;106:823–7.
33. Attinger CE, Evans KK, Bulan E, et al. Angiosomes of the foot and ankle and clinical implications for limb salvage: reconstruction, incisions, and revascularization. Plast Reconstr Surg 2006;117:261S–93S.
34. Kwan MK, Merican AM, Ahmad TS. Reconstruction of the heel defect with in-step island flap. A report of four cases. Med J Malaysia 2005;60:S104–7.
35. Butler CE, Chevray P. Retrograde-flow medial plantar island flap reconstruction of distal forefoot, toe, and webspace defects. Ann Plast Surg 2002;49:196–201.
36. Zgonis T, Stapleton JJ, Papakostas I. Local and distant pedicle flaps for soft tissue reconstruction of the diabetic foot: a stepwise approach with the use of external fixation. In: Zgonis T, editor. Surgical reconstruction of the diabetic foot and ankle. Philadelphia: Lippincott, Williams & Wilkins; 2009. p. 170–92.
37. Zgonis T, Stapleton JJ. Innovative techniques in preventing and salvaging neurovascular pedicle flaps in reconstructive foot and ankle surgery. Foot Ankle Spec 2008;1:97–104.
38. Cigna E, Fioramonti P, Fino P, et al. Island lateral plantar artery perforator flap for reconstruction of weight-bearing plantar areas. Foot Ankle Surg 2011;17:e13–6.
39. Ramanujam CL, Zgonis T. Primary arthrodesis and sural artery flap coverage for subtalar joint osteomyelitis in a diabetic patient. Clin Podiatr Med Surg 2011;28: 421–7.
40. Ahn DK, Lew DH, Roh TS, et al. Reconstruction of ankle and heel defects with peroneal artery perforator-based pedicled flaps. Arch Plast Surg 2015;42: 619–25.
41. Bekara F, Herlin C, Mojallal A, et al. A systematic review and meta-analysis of perforator-pedicled propeller flaps in lower extremity defects: identification of risk factors for complications. Plast Reconstr Surg 2016;137:314–31.
42. Innocenti M, Menichini G, Baldrighi C, et al. Are there risk factors for complications of perforator-based propeller flaps for lower-extremity reconstruction? Clin Orthop Relat Res 2014;472:2276–86.
43. Kallio M, Vikatmaa P, Kantonen I, et al. Strategies for free flap transfer and revascularisation with long-term outcome in the treatment of large diabetic foot lesions. Eur J Vasc Endovasc Surg 2015;50:223–30.
44. Lee YK, Park KY, Koo YT, et al. Analysis of multiple risk factors affecting the result of free flap transfer for necrotising soft tissue defects of the lower extremities in patients with type 2 diabetes mellitus. J Plast Reconstr Aesthet Surg 2014;67: 624–8.
45. Oznur A, Zgonis T. Closure of major diabetic foot wounds and defects with external fixation. Clin Podiatr Med Surg 2007;24:519–28.
46. Ramanujam CL, Facaros Z, Zgonis T. Abductor hallucis muscle flap with circular external fixation for Charcot foot osteomyelitis: a case report. Diabet Foot Ankle 2012;2. http://dx.doi.org/10.3402/dfa.v2i0.6336.
47. Ramanujam CL, Facaros Z, Zgonis T. External fixation for surgical off-loading of diabetic soft tissue reconstruction. Clin Podiatr Med Surg 2011;28:211–6.

Revisional Surgery of the Diabetic Charcot Foot and Ankle

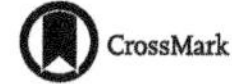

Patrick R. Burns, DPM[a,b,*], Spencer J. Monaco, DPM[b]

KEYWORDS

- Charcot neuroarthropathy • Revisional foot and ankle surgery
- Tibiotalocalcaneal arthrodesis • Superconstruct • Ilizarov external fixation
- Diabetes mellitus

KEY POINTS

- Revision of Charcot neuroarthropathy (CN) requires proper workup, including vascular status, nutritional status, laboratory studies, including blood glucose control, and inflammatory markers to ensure success.
- Osteomyelitis must be ruled out or managed appropriately for revision CN surgery success.
- The theory of a "superconstruct" should be understood to guide preparation and fixation concepts during CN reconstruction and revision.
- Arthrodesis is a large part of revision surgery for CN and, including the rearfoot and ankle, may be beneficial for controlling the deformity and biomechanical forces, in a "pan-fusion" concept.

INTRODUCTION

Charcot neuroarthropathy (CN) is potentially one of the most challenging conditions that a foot and ankle specialist may encounter. Studies have shown that patients affected with CN demonstrate a lower quality of life when compared with patients without CN.[1,2] In some cases, the condition can be treated nonoperatively without the need for surgical intervention.[3] Nonoperative management includes accommodative footwear, orthotics, and/or bracing. Surgical intervention may be warranted when instability, deformity, and a nonplantigrade foot can no longer be controlled with these nonoperative measures. The resultant CN deformities may leave the patient at risk for ulceration that is unable to heal, potentially leading to an infection and amputation.

Disclosure Statement: The authors have nothing to disclose.
[a] University of Pittsburgh School of Medicine, Pittsburgh, PA, USA; [b] UPMC Podiatric Medicine and Surgery Residency, Pittsburgh, PA, USA
* Corresponding author. 1515 Locust Street, #350, Pittsburgh, PA 15219.
E-mail address: burnsp@upmc.edu

Clin Podiatr Med Surg 34 (2017) 77–92
http://dx.doi.org/10.1016/j.cpm.2016.07.009
podiatric.theclinics.com

Long-standing deformities whereby the CN process has consolidated the foot or ankle in maligned position can be extremely daunting and difficult to correct to a more anatomic position. Index reconstruction may include exostectomies, osteotomies, and arthrodesis with varying forms of fixation. Research has demonstrated that patients with uncontrolled diabetes mellitus and peripheral neuropathy have higher rates of surgical complications when compared with patients with uncomplicated diabetes mellitus and nondiabetics.[4] If the primary attempt at reconstruction fails, the complexity of the surgery increases. Functional limb preservation/limb salvage versus major amputation becomes of critical importance for the overall well-being of the patient. Revisional surgery should be individualized to each patient and each case should be comprehensively evaluated. This article reviews how to evaluate these difficult cases to maximize the opportunity for a successful revision surgery. Principles of treating unstable CN deformities with ulcerations and infection, superconstructs, and current accepted techniques are discussed.

COMPREHENSIVE PREOPERATIVE WORKUP

Each patient undergoing revision should be optimized from a systemic and local standpoint. Consultation with an endocrinologist, nutritionist, and a vascular surgeon can help correct any insufficiencies if present. Patients should be optimized for both long-term and short-term blood glucose control. Preoperative blood glucose greater than 200 mg/dL and a hemoglobin A1C (HbA1c) greater than 8% have been found to place these patients at a higher risk of surgical site infection and other complications such as nonunion.[5] These parameters should be monitored before any major surgery in this patient population, but in particular need to be addressed for any attempt at revision. Although patients with CN typically have "bounding pulses" as thought of in the vascular theory of the disease, it is clear that the presence of pulses is not itself indicative of adequate blood flow.[6] Noninvasive arterial studies such as ankle brachial index, toe brachial index, toe pressures, and waveforms can extremely beneficial to help identify a patient with macrovascular and/or microvascular disease. Consults to vascular surgery should be considered so there can be a determination on intervention. If this has not already been completed for the index procedure, it is particularly important in the setting of revision.

Unfortunately, many patients with CN have an increased body mass index, but this does not always correlate to the actual nutrition of the patient. Routine laboratory testing such as vitamin D, albumin, prealbumin, and leukocyte counts before reconstruction can identify any nutritional abnormalities.[7] Nutrition consults and supplements are not only required for those with wound issues but also in this population in general and should be a standard consideration.

In the face of an open ulceration, known history of infection, or nonunion, obtaining serum inflammatory markers such as erythrocyte sedimentation rate (ESR) and C-reactive protein (CRP) along with a complete blood count can aid in the diagnosis of osteomyelitis.[8,9] These laboratory tests can be a useful adjunct to clinical findings as well as intraoperative cultures and frozen sections. Individuals who have a smoking or chewing tobacco history should be counseled on the deleterious effects of active nicotine use on soft tissue and bone healing, and a cessation program should be implemented.[10] In order to optimize attempt at successful reconstruction, factors that are modifiable should be addressed before surgical intervention (**Box 1**).

Last, but not least, consideration should be given to the social aspects of the treatment process. Patients undergoing large revision surgeries require prolonged non-weight-bearing (NWB), which requires assistance in daily living. Without a good

Box 1
Preoperative workup for the diabetic patient with Charcot neuroarthropathy

- Noninvasive arterial studies (ankle brachial index, toe brachial index, toe pressures, waveforms, transcutaneous oxygen pressures)
- Complete blood count
- Basic metabolic panel
- Albumin and prealbumin
- Vitamin D
- Hemoglobin A1c
- C-reactive protein
- Erythrocyte sedimentation rate

support system, it is difficult for the patient to comply with postoperative protocols like NWB. Short-term care facilities should be considered for rehabilitation. These facilities can aid the patient in their daily needs, their weight-bearing status, dressing changes, antibiotic delivery, safe transfers, and transportation.

UNDERSTANDING WHY THE INDEX PROCEDURE FAILED

In the setting of revision, it is important to evaluate the entire problem, and this requires obtaining as much information as possible about the initial presentation, workup, and medical and surgical treatment. This information can aid in the understanding of the current problem and help create a holistic approach for future reconstruction and treatment.

If an ulceration or infection was present previously, was the treatment appropriate? Did the patient have antibiotics, and if so, were they oral or intravenous (IV). What was the offending pathogen? The findings give insight into the extent of the infection, and if soft tissue or bone was involved. Were cultures taken? Were they intraoperative bone cultures or superficial swabs of the skin? The management of infection may not have been worked up, treated, or eradicated fully. Complete understanding of infection and location is imperative before the start of any reconstruction.

Reviewing the preoperative radiographs and index procedure constructs can provide valuable information to potentially why the reconstruction failed. Certain types of CN are more unstable and more difficult to treat, such as the case with deformities involving the talonavicular and ankle joints. The hardware chosen for the first reconstruction may not have been sufficient to withstand the deforming forces of the CN, thus leading to failure. Not only should one consider where the hardware was placed, but also the type of fixation and technique. Cannulated versus solid screws, titanium versus stainless, locking versus nonlocking, and orientation can give insight as to potential reasons for failure. Index fixation can be addressed during the revision by understanding proper Arbeitsgemeinschaft für Osteosynthesefragen techniques and the subtle differences between the types of fixation.

ADDRESSING THE ISSUES DURING CHARCOT NEUROARTHROPATHY REVISION

Infection

Whether infection was present at the initial surgery or at the time of revision, it must be managed to have any success of salvage. As mentioned earlier, proper laboratory values must be obtained. It is important to have the expertise of infectious disease specialties. The surgeon must be aware of the laboratory values and coordinate a team approach. The radiographic changes of CN and infection may be overlapping and thus challenging the overall clinical picture.

A staged protocol is typically executed in the setting of possible osteomyelitis. Previous hardware is removed and fresh frozen section and bone biopsy are performed.[11] It is important to document and communicate to the consulting services the intraoperative findings, such as presence of purulence, location of biopsy, and the overall quality of the bone. With proper cultures, the patient can receive pathogen-specific IV antibiotic therapy, which can be augmented with broad spectrum heat stabile local antibiotics. Polymethylmethacrylate (PMMA) is a traditional method of delivery, but other types of beads can be used such as absorbable (**Fig. 1**). At the authors' institution, PMMA are preferred due to the increased drainage observed with absorbable beads. The PMMA spacer can easily be removed during the second operation (**Fig. 2**A). In order to maintain skeletal stabilization, typically an external fixation is used such as a circular ring external fixator.[12] This device allows for not only stabilization of the deformity but also continued monitoring of the soft tissue envelope and ulceration management (**Fig. 2**B). Obtaining clean soft tissue and bone cultures, healing ulcerations, and surgical removal of osteomyelitis will provide the optimal conditions for a successful CN revision surgery.

Soft Tissue

The triceps surae complex has been implicated in much abnormality of the foot and ankle. An equinus contracture has been shown to be a deforming force causing increased pressure across the plantar midfoot and forefoot with reference to patients with diabetes mellitus and neuropathic ulcerations.[13] The deforming force must be addressed appropriately. Lengthening of the Achilles tendon traditionally in this population has been performed through percutaneous tendo-Achilles lengthening (TAL) (**Fig. 3**). Several studies originally showed the offloading potential of this procedure but may not be the panacea once thought.[14–16] Based on benchmark research, many surgeons performed a percutaneous TAL in conjunction with CN reconstruction. More recently, it has been learned that following this procedure the Achilles tendon regains its strength, and the ankle continues to lose motion several months later. The continued contracture may be one of the reasons failure occurred following the

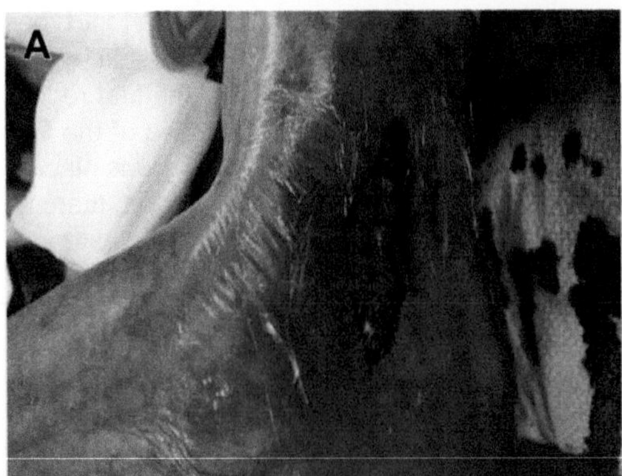

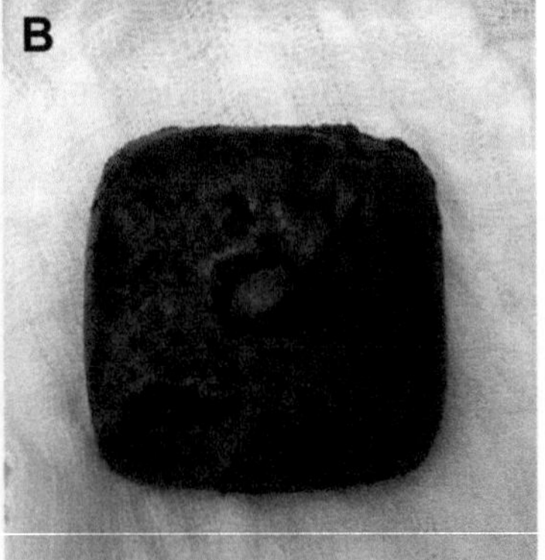

Fig. 1. PMMA beads (*A*) and single spacer (*B*) typical for local antibiotic delivery in revision salvage.

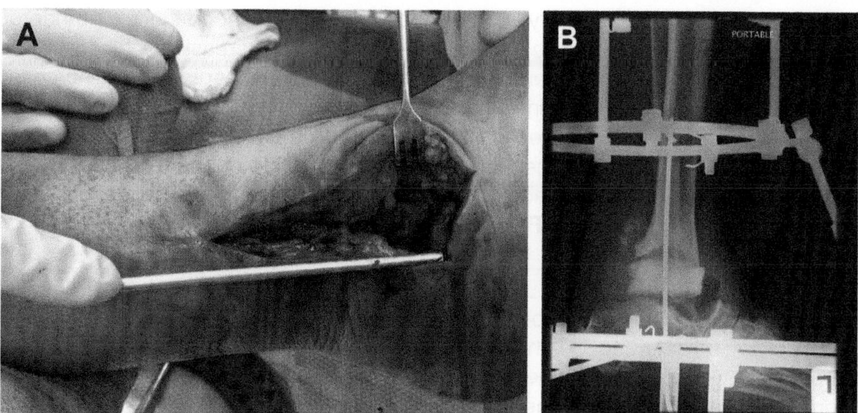

Fig. 2. Intraoperative picture of a typical lateral ankle incision, showing the PMMA spacer (*A*) and radiograph (*B*) showing typical placement during staged ankle reconstruction and revision.

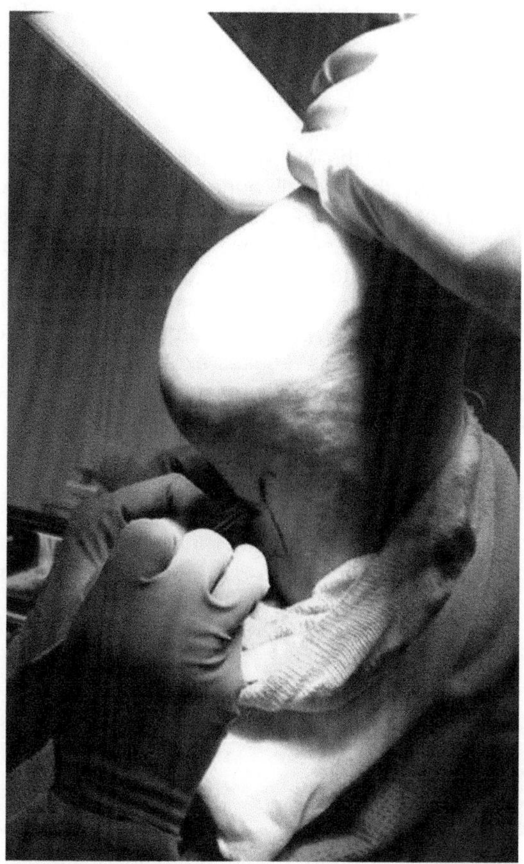

Fig. 3. Typical percutaneous TAL used in CN.

index reconstruction. Potentially, the Achilles tendon itself continues to undergo changes secondary to the disease process, becoming increasingly glycosylated. Percutaneous TAL has also been shown to be less stable, leading to an increased amount of ruptures, tendinosis in the watershed area, calcaneal gait, or plantar heel ulceration.[17] During revision, the Achilles contracture must be taken into consideration. A more proximal gastrocnemius recession may lend to better results in overall lengthening of the posterior muscle groups as well as have a more permanent effect on power and range of motion (**Fig. 4**).[17,18]

Bone

After a consolidated CN event, bone fragmentation, fracture, dislocation, and subsequent deformity seem to be the overwhelming concern. All the previous issues addressed are important, but clearly the bony architecture is a foremost worry. The deformed skeletal anatomy is the major source of the pressure that plagues most of these patients, which makes it a top priority. The deformity planning relies on radiographs and bone abnormality. Adequate bone must be resected during revision to correct deformity and remove any undue tension on the soft tissue envelope. As discussed before, the presence of all osteomyelitis must be resected. In some cases, angular deformities are addressed with removal of an appropriate wedge depending on which planes are affected. Deformity correction can be either in the midfoot or the ankle and should be templated before the start of the revision. The result of wedge resections is multiple. First, it makes a more plantigrade and rectus foot or ankle. It also allows for reduction of tension on the overlying skin to prevent or aid in the healing of any ulcerations. This concept is a principle of "superconstructs" popularized by Sammarco (**Figs. 5** and **6**).[19]

Finally, one must also consider the integrity of the bone. As stated previously, there are physiologic issues with the overall bone quality in this group of patients. Exchanging hardware is not only complicated by this, but also previous fixation constructs increase the local weakness of the bone and decreases the quality needed for new fixation. Considerations have to be made to extend beyond the zone of injury to gain stability and access new areas of potentially stronger bone, which were not previously affected by the CN event or previous hardware. In some cases where the deformity is affecting the midfoot, this requires extending arthrodesis to all columns and even the subtalar joint to adequately control the deforming forces. In select cases, the ankle joint must be included as well.

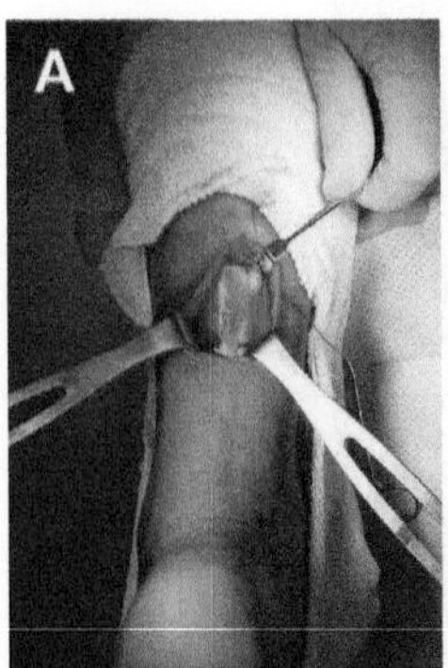

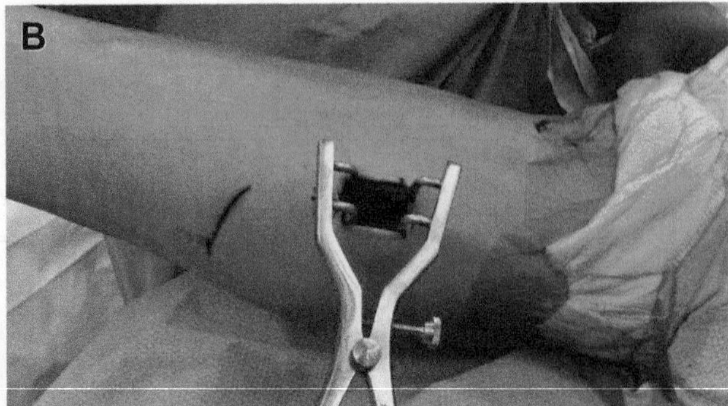

Fig. 4. Open posterior Strayer-type gastrocnemius recession (*A*) and more proximal medial Baumann type (*B*).

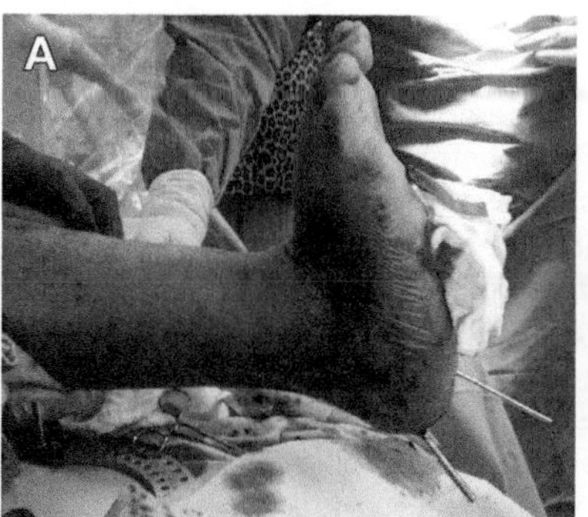

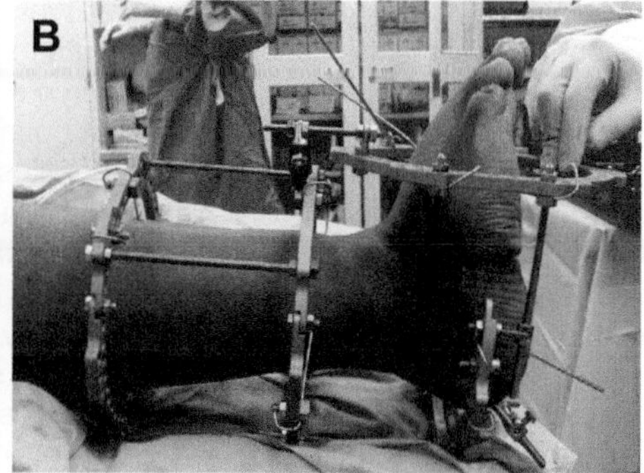

Fig. 5. Midfoot CN with chronic wound and osteomyelitis. Note the dorsiflexed rocker-bottom deformity (*A*) and the correction after osteotomy (*B*). Note the amount of wrinkle and midfoot deformity reduction taking tension from the plantar foot, which aids in healing.

Hardware

The type and utilization of hardware in patients with CN, and in particular during revision, are one of the most controversial topics. Patients with diabetic neuropathy cannot be treated with the same techniques as those without neuropathy. As discussed earlier, this can be due to numerous factors. In the setting of CN in patients with diabetes mellitus, there can be both local osteopenia secondary to the disease process but also systemic complications related to renal disease as it pertains to the homeostasis of calcium.[20] The revision patient may also be many months into previous treatment

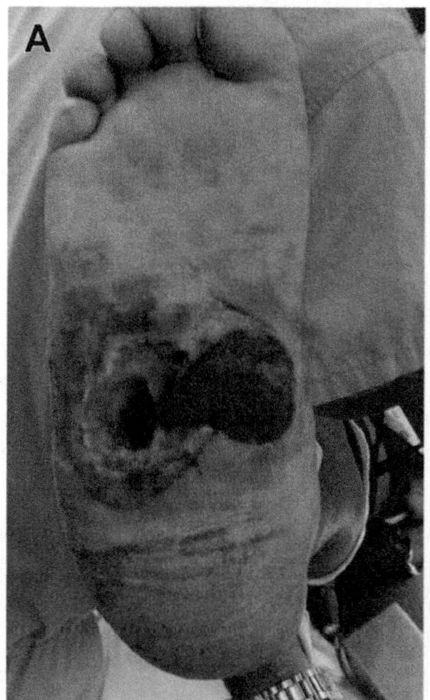

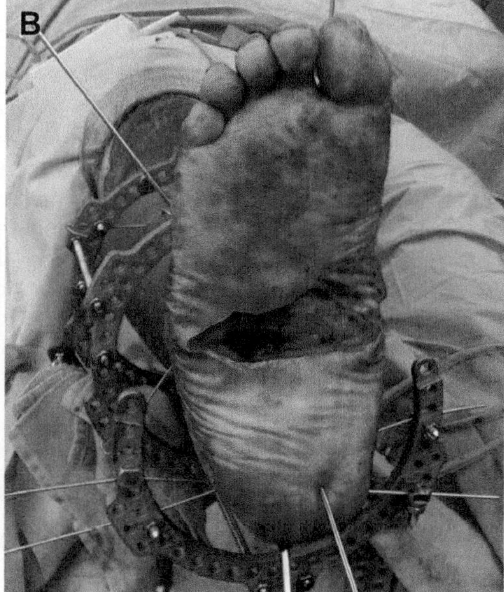

Fig. 6. The same revision surgery for CN. The patient had prior bone exostectomy. Note the continued wound and prior free flap (*A*), and amount of reduction in tension, the amount of wrinkle plantar (*B*) after revision osteotomy, and deformity reduction.

with potentially prolonged periods of NWB resulting in local disuse osteopenia. Disuse osteopenia creates the perfect environment for compromised bone, making adequate fixation even more challenging. Sammarco's "superconstruct" principles may lend valuable guidelines in achieving the most optimal construct (**Box 2**).

The problems with fixation for CN deformities are numerous. First, the soft tissue envelope limits the size and position of the hardware that can be used. In certain cases, an ulcer may be present due to the inability to be healed before the start of revision. Second, the size and shape of the foot and ankle bones are a limiting factor. Anatomy becomes even more difficult in the setting of CN, whereby deformed or missing bones are present due to the Charcot process and certainly in situation of previous surgery, osseous wedge resection may have been attempted. The soft tissue envelope and bony architecture make applying quality stable fixation in the best mechanical area a demanding task.

A decision must be made about the type of fixation to be used. There is no clear consensus whether internal or external fixation is superior. At times, it is a combination through a staged protocol, depending on coinciding factors like osteomyelitis and the presence of ulceration. Certainly the strongest fixation tolerated by the location, bone quality, and skin envelope is recommended. General fixation selections to add strength tend to be larger solid screws and locked plates. With the advent of anatomic plates, this allows for more options as to orientation and location versus traditional plating. Intramedullary (IM) fixation may be more mechanically stable but not practical in all situations. IM constructs such as axial screw fixation can be used through beaming the columns of the foot. This technique however still allows for rotational moments, so it may be necessary to "lock the beam" with a locking plate (**Fig. 7**). IM fixation can also be used to control hindfoot and ankle deforming forces. External fixation is an option; however, it certainly has complications. Unfortunately, no cases are exactly the same, and the decisions on type of fixation have to be individualized. There are similarities between deformities, but CN tends to be variable in the location, deformity produced, presence of infection, and prior surgeries performed.

LOCATION OF DEFORMITY

Reconstruction of a CN deformity requires complete understanding of the location of the deformity. It seems that midfoot CN deformities may be more common and stable in general, whereas rearfoot/ankle deformities become more unstable and require surgical intervention. Because of the issues of instability and the degree of CN deformity, it potentially has a higher likelihood to fail reconstruction. When revising a midfoot CN, one must consider the location within the foot (Lisfranc or midtarsal) and remember the forces carried through this area. As the apex of deformity moves more proximally toward the rearfoot and ankle, the deforming forces increase, which stresses the affected area and any fixation construct applied. Simply performing a posterior muscle group lengthening in conjuncture with column beaming may not be enough to reduce

Box 2
The superconstruct concept for the diabetic patient with Charcot neuroarthropathy

- Resect enough bone to allow reduction of deformity and reduce skin tension
- Extend fixation/arthrodesis beyond the "zone of injury"
- Use the strongest devices, in the most mechanically sound way tolerated by local anatomy
- Use the strongest fixation devices permitted by local skin and soft tissue

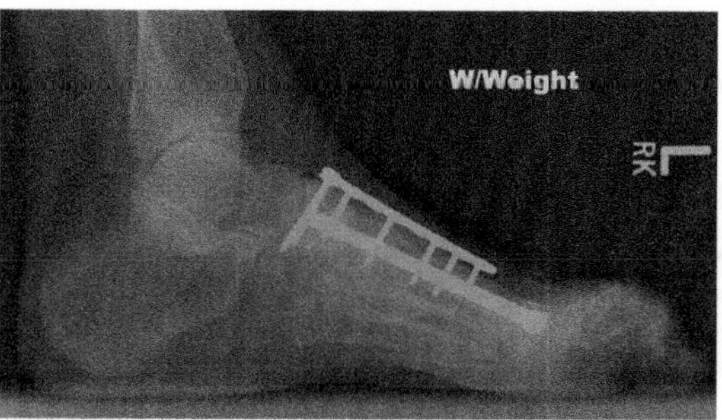

Fig. 7. Radiographic example of "locking the beam" for medial column arthrodesis, to combat potential rotational forces allowed by beam technique alone.

these forces (**Fig. 8**). Consideration should be given into including a subtalar and/or ankle arthrodesis in selective midfoot and rearfoot reconstructions, and in particular, revision. The "pan-foot" construct can aid in negated these deforming forces such as the equinus contracture and help redistribute the overall load from the patients weight up the leg (**Fig. 9**). The technique of "backwards beaming" allows for controlling the deforming forces more proximal to the deformity and extends past the zone of injury, which allows for a more mechanically sound fixation construct.

CASE EXAMPLES

Case 1

A patient with a history of diabetes mellitus, diabetic neuropathy, and a trimalleolar ankle fracture with subsequent open reduction and internal fixation continued to have edema with progressing deformity (**Fig. 10**A). On initial presentation, she had increased temperature to the right ankle, instability with varus/valgus stress, and obvious clinical deformity. Her radiographs clearly showed destructive changes to the ankle with a varus deformity (**Fig. 10**B, C). She clearly had CN changes with concern of possible infection as well. She had no history of wound complications but white blood cell count (WBC) of 11.3, elevated CRP 4.2, and ESR of 110.

Discussion was made about possible conversion to arthrodesis after removal of hardware, bone biopsy, and soft tissue frozen section. Consent was also made for a staged protocol with external fixation depending on intraoperative findings. Intraoperatively, immediate purulent material was identified (**Fig. 10**D). The hardware was removed; the bone was debrided to what appeared healthy (**Fig. 10**E), and the void was filled with an antibiotic spacer (**Fig. 10**F). Cultures were obtained; the ankle

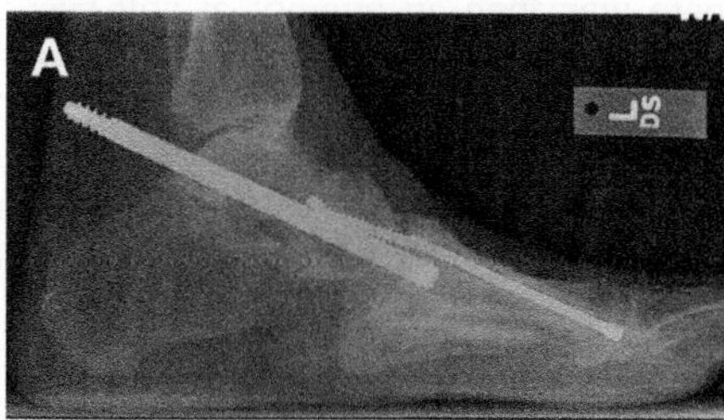

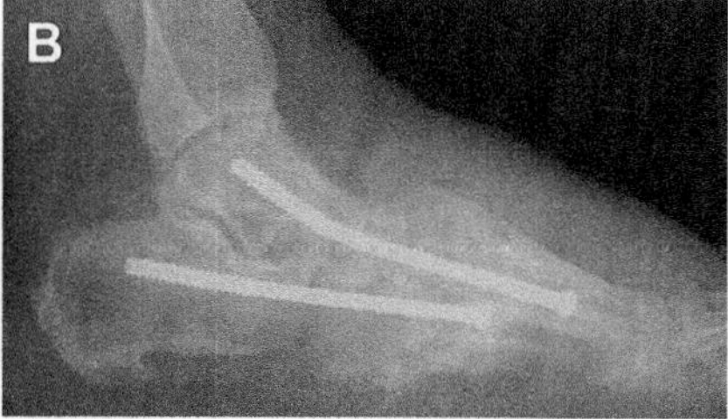

Fig. 8. Medial column beam technique failure example with migration (*A*) and fracture of hardware (*B*).

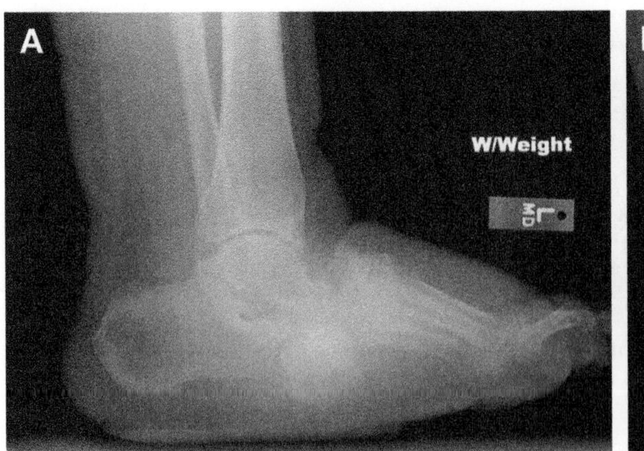

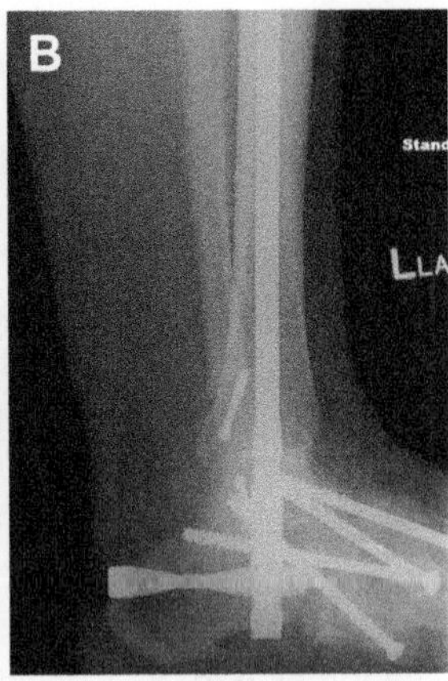

Fig. 9. Example of significant CN of the midfoot, with typical equinus and multiple levels of deformity (*A*) surgically corrected with a global fusion to address and correct all issues (*B*).

was reduced and then held in place with an external fixator (**Fig. 10**G). The external fixator maintained alignment and stability during the coming months. The patient followed with infectious disease and had appropriate antibiotics (**Fig. 10**H, I). Laboratory values were followed, and once normalized, decision was made to perform the definitive surgery.

The external fixator was removed in the clinical setting and a cast applied. All wounds were healed, and over the following 2 weeks, the external fixator pins sites were allowed to heal, before the definitive surgery. The antibiotic spacer and transarticular pins were left in place (**Fig. 10**J). The patient then returned to the operating room. The spacer was removed, and new cultures and frozen sections were taken. With normal laboratory values and no WBC on the frozen section, the patient was converted to a tibiotalocalcaneal arthrodesis with allograft and IM fixation (**Fig. 10**K, L).

The patient was kept NWB for 10 weeks, transferred to a Charcot restraint orthotic walker (CROW) for 6 months, and then upright bracing on custom shoes until 1 year (**Fig. 10**M, N) without wounds or deformity.

Case 2

A patient was referred to the authors' institution with a history of diabetes mellitus, diabetic neuropathy, and increasing CN deformity. There were original issues with the lateral column and a wound at the fifth metatarsal. The patient had a partial fifth ray amputation, which healed the original wound but had continued instability and preulcerative areas now at the lateral ankle. There was then an attempt at soft tissue balancing to address the deformity. The patient healed the surgical wound, but there continued to be edema, instability, and deformity. He was unbraceable and developed wounds lateral at the malleolus and plantar lateral heel (**Fig. 11**A). Every attempt, including total contact casting, was exhausted, with no change. Over the past months from the casting, he developed wounds to the tips of the remaining toes as well (**Fig. 11**B).

His radiographs clearly showed progressive significant bone destruction, chronic changes to the calcaneus, tibia, and almost complete dissolution of the talus. The varus deformity and instability were obvious as well (**Fig. 11**C, D). Laboratory values were ordered with elevated CRP 7.3 and ESR of 97, but a normal WBC.

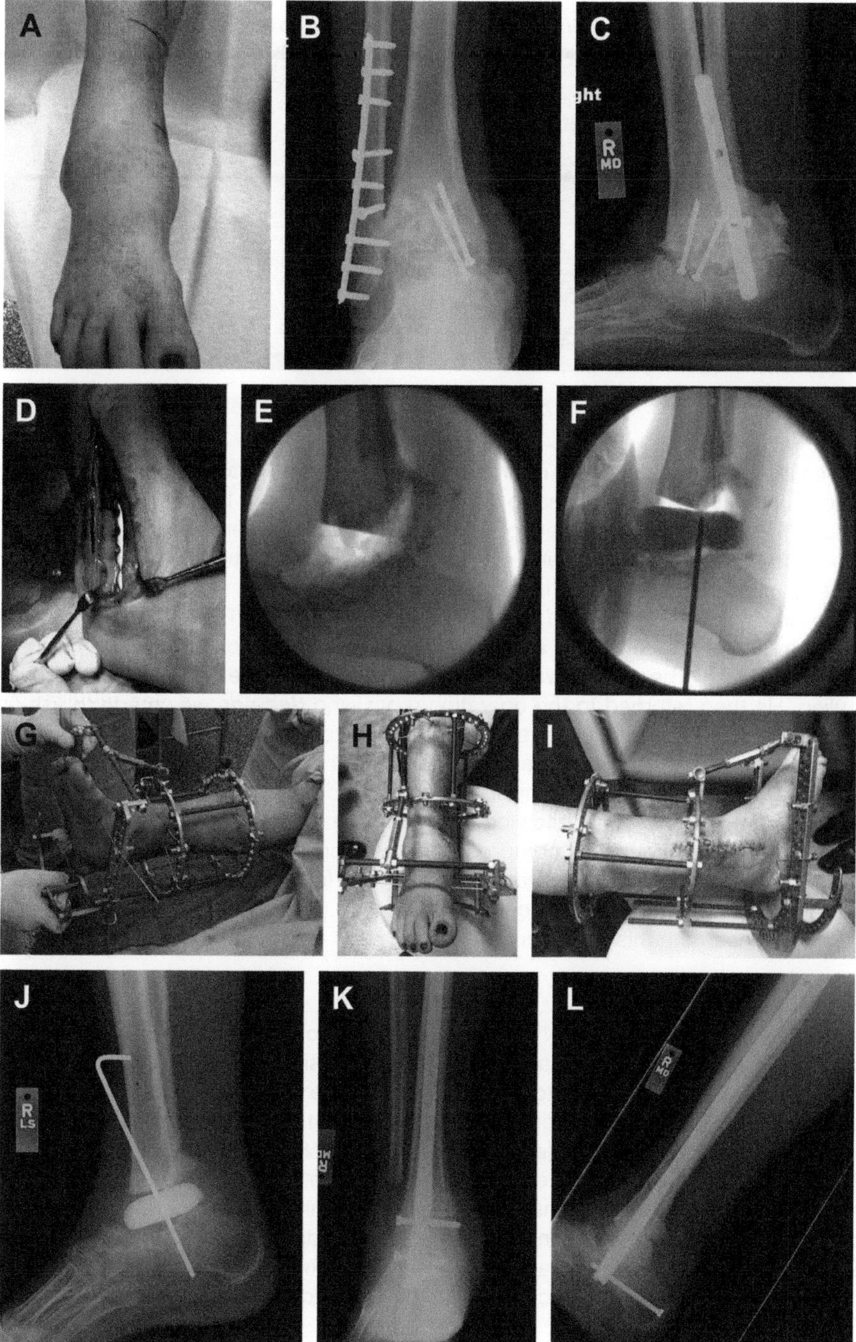

Fig. 10. (*A–N*) Staged reconstruction of a CN with concomitant osteomyelitis.

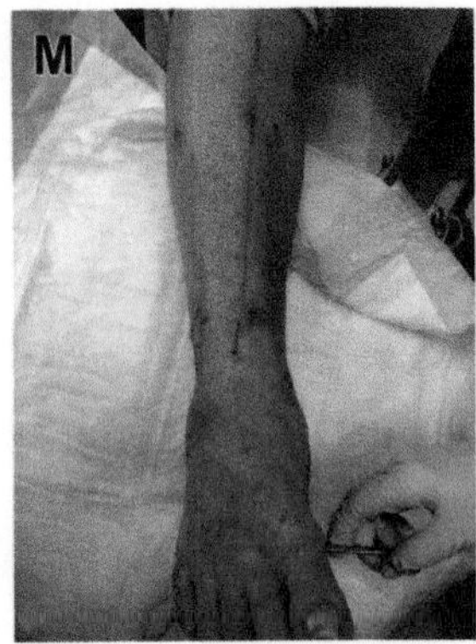

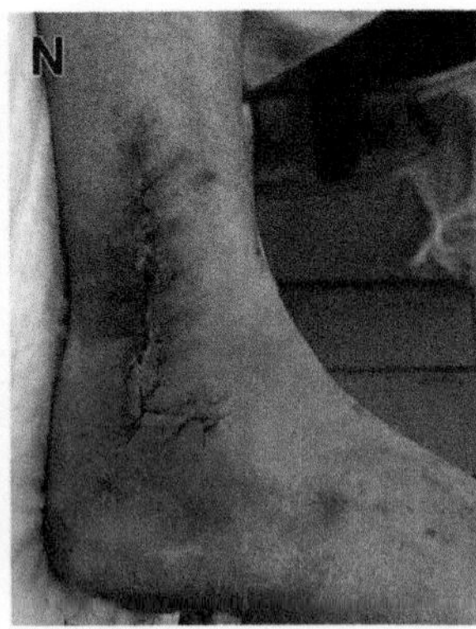

Fig. 10. (*continued*).

The patient was taken to the operating room, and an osteotomy was performed to remove unhealthy bone and also to address the deformity for later reconstruction attempts (**Fig. 11**E, F). Frozen sections and cultures were taken; an antibiotic spacer was placed to fill the void, and an external fixator was applied to hold reduction, maintain alignment, and aid in soft tissue healing (**Fig. 11**G, H).

The external fixator remained for approximately 10 weeks (**Fig. 11**I, J). During that time, the patient finished his IV antibiotic therapy and laboratory test values returned to normal limits. The fixator was removed in the clinical setting, and a cast was applied. He then returned to the operating room, and decision was made to use an anterior incision to avoid the previous wounds laterally. The bone was prepared, and frozen sections taken and deemed "clean" with 1 WBC/hpf. An allograft was fashioned for the void, and an anterior plate was applied (**Fig. 11**K). This technique gave the best attempt at fixation, allowing fixation in the tuberosity because the anterior portion of the calcaneus was compromised and would not likely hold an IM device. He was NWB for 3 months, transitioned to a CROW for 6 months, and then to upright bracing on his custom shoes without issue (**Fig. 11**L). The upright bracing may be permanent in cases like this to protect the construct.

Case 3

A patient was referred with a CN event in the left midfoot. It was monitored and treated nonsurgically for several months. He was casted, transitioned into a boot, and using a knee roller. Initially he seemed to consolidate but once he was transitioned to custom shoes, he noticed increased redness and edema again. He seemed to start a new CN event with progressive changes on plain radiographs through the Lisfranc area (**Fig. 12**A, B). He was also developing a preulcerative area medially, and a decision was made to undertake reconstruction through arthrodesis (**Fig. 12**C). During his follow-up, the patient had continued edema and mild discomfort. He was transitioned slowly over several months to a CROW and then bracing. His radiographs began to show issues with nonunion, increasing deformity, and progressive hardware failure (**Fig. 12**D, E).

He had no open wounds or issues with wound healing during his prior surgery, and an HbA1c of 7.2. He then had a small preulcerative area plantar lateral subcuboid with typical rocker-bottom appearance (**Fig. 12**F, G). He had obvious failure of hardware, and decision was made for revision surgery. This time, his ankle would be included. Originally, he had first and second column along with subtalar joint arthrodesis to

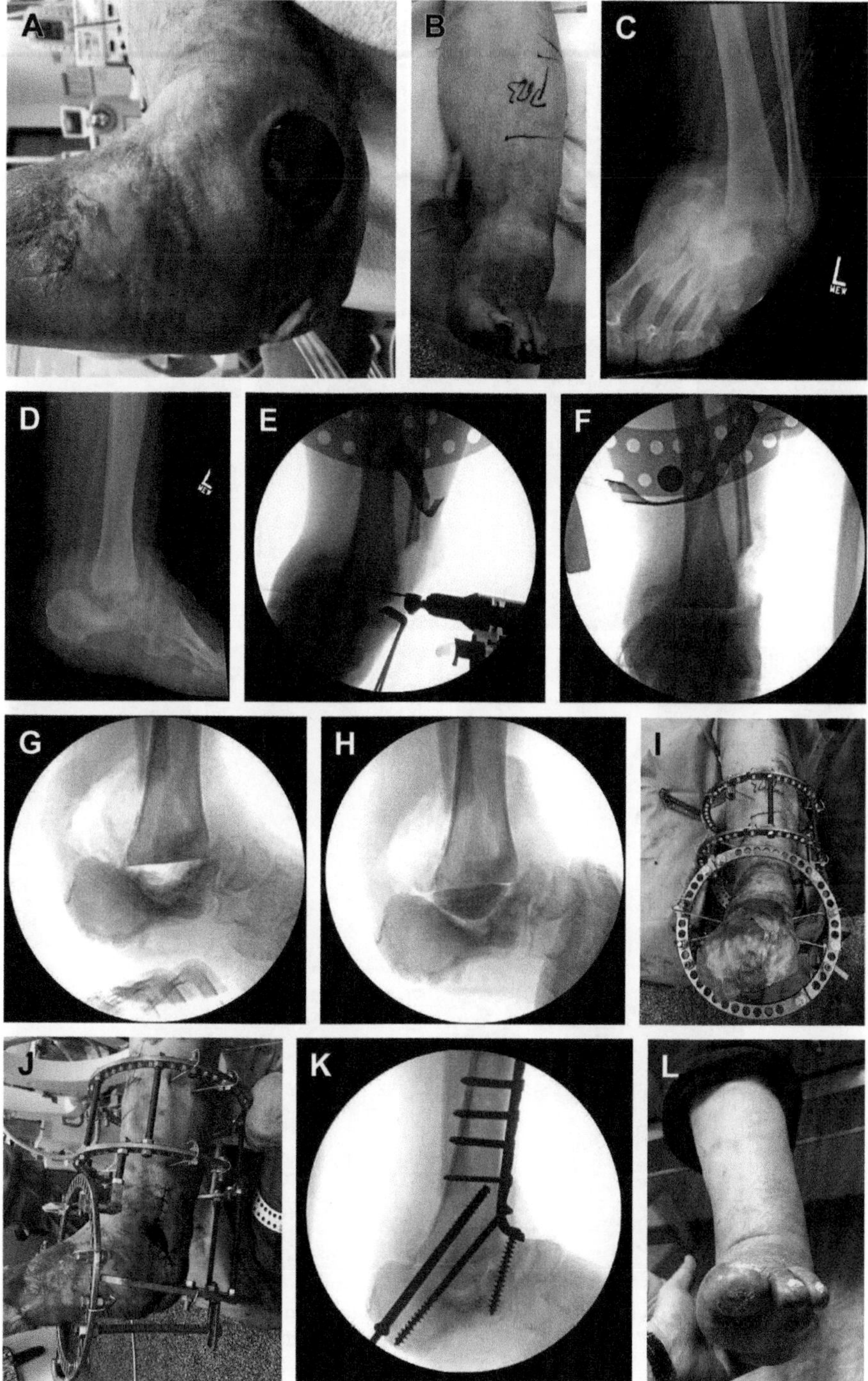

Fig. 11. (*A–L*) Staged reconstruction of an unstable varus ankle with CN and prior fifth ray amputation.

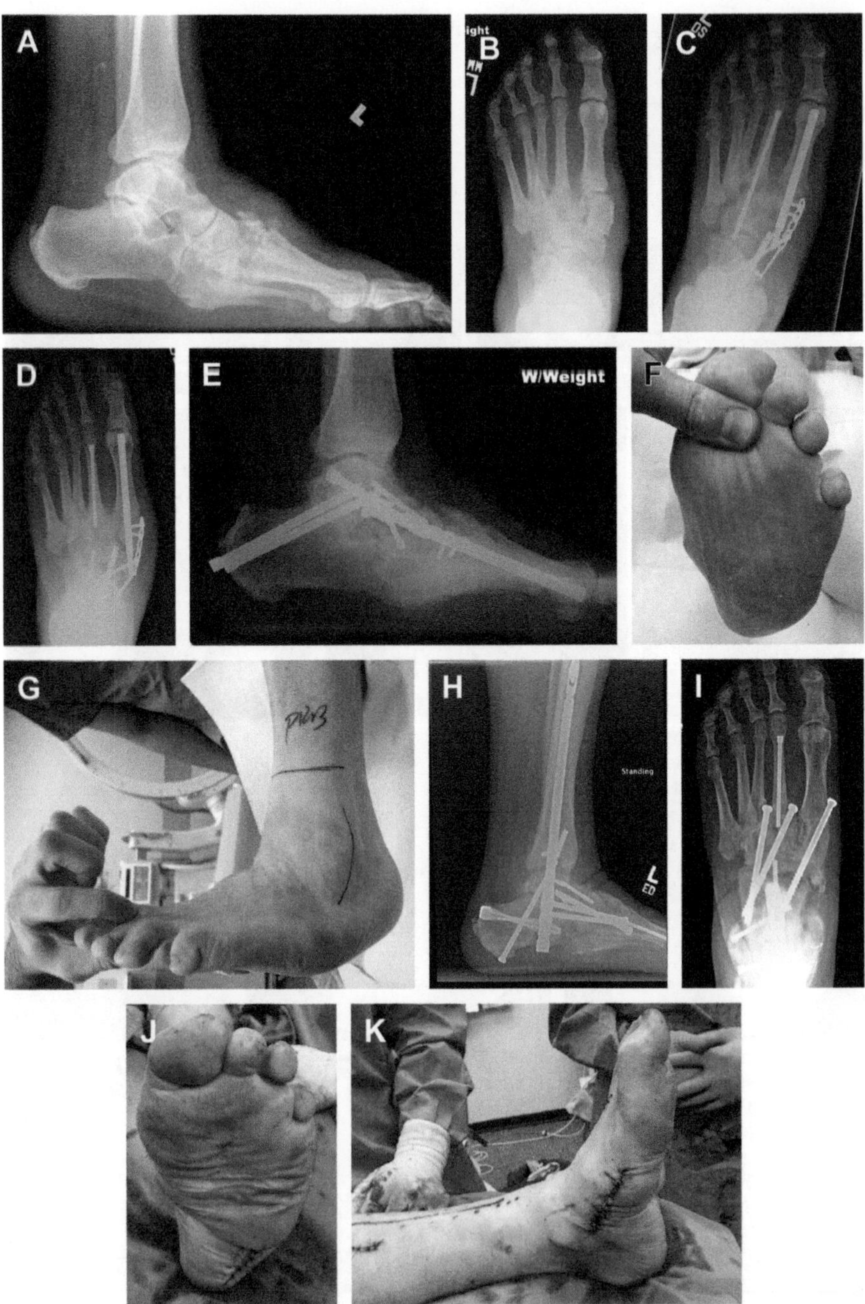

Fig. 12. (*A–K*) Staged revision of a midfoot CN that failed original arthrodesis and then converted to a "pan-fusion" to correct and control the deformity.

try to control deformity forces and stresses. He now had continued issues and preulcerative lateral column lesion.

He was taken to the operating room, where most of the hardware was removed and revision "pan-fusion" was performed. The ankle was included through a lateral approach, allowing access to the distal fibular for autograft (**Fig. 12**H, I). After reduction and correction, there was a more "normal" appearance to the arch, with tension removed plantarly as noted by postoperative skin wrinkling at the plantar aspect (**Fig. 12**J, K).

The patient healed all wounds with less edema and discomfort. He transitioned to a CROW around 3 months and then bracing several months later. He continues with an ankle foot orthosis-type brace because it helps him "mentally" know there is issue with the left leg but clinically and radiographically is stable without hardware issues. Including the ankle as a "pan-fusion" for recurrence, plantar lateral wounds, or CN that involves proximal to the Lisfranc joint seems to be a useful tool at the authors' institution for diabetic limb salvage.

SUMMARY

Reconstruction, in particular revision, in patients with diabetic CN deformity whether midfoot or ankle is an extremely daunting task for foot and ankle specialists. Comprehensively evaluating each case requires an individualized approach to meet each patient's needs. Before the start of any reconstruction or revision, the social aspects must be taken into consideration. A comprehensive workup, including noninvasive arterial studies and appropriate laboratory tests to address any insufficiencies or ongoing infections, must not be overlooked. Complete understandings of why the index reconstruction failed will assist in developing a treatment plan. Last, using techniques such as superconstructs and using the most stable construct possible to negate deforming forces will provide the surgeon with the best chance at a successful revision operation.

REFERENCES

1. Dhawan V, Spratt KF, Pinzur MS, et al. Reliability of AOFAS diabetic foot questionnaire in Charcot arthropathy: stability, internal consistency, and measurable difference. Foot Ankle Int 2005;26:717–31.
2. Raspovic KM, Wukich DK. Self-reported quality of life in patients with diabetes: a comparison of patients with and without Charcot neuroarthropathy. Foot Ankle Int 2014;35:195–200.
3. Pinzur MS. Neutral ring fixation for high-risk nonplantigrade Charcot midfoot deformity. Foot Ankle Int 2007;28:961–6.
4. Wukich DK, McMillen RL, Lowery NJ, et al. Surgical site infections after foot and ankle surgery: a comparison of patients with and without diabetes. Diabetes Care 2011;34:2211–3.
5. Wukich DK, Crim BE, Frykberg RG, et al. Neuropathy and poorly controlled diabetes increase the rate of surgical site infection after foot and ankle surgery. J Bone Joint Surg Am 2014;96:832–9.
6. Schaper NC, Andros G, Apelqvist J, et al. Specific guidelines for the diagnosis and treatment of peripheral arterial disease in a patient with diabetes and ulceration of the foot 2011. Diabetes Metab Res Rev 2012;28(Suppl 1):236–7.
7. Pinzur MS, Sage R, Stuck R, et al. Transcutaneous oxygen as a predictor of wound healing in amputations of the foot and ankle. Foot Ankle Int 1992;13:271–2.

8. Kaleta JL, Fleischli JW, Reilly CH. The diagnosis of osteomyelitis in diabetes using erythrocyte sedimentation rate: a pilot study. J Am Podiatr Med Assoc 2001;91: 445–50.
9. Fleischer AE, Didyk AA, Woods JB, et al. Combined clinical and laboratory testing improves diagnostic accuracy for osteomyelitis in the diabetic foot. J Foot Ankle Surg 2009;48:39–46.
10. Raikin SM, Landsman JC, Alexander VA, et al. Effect of nicotine on the rate and strength of long bone fracture healing. Clin Orthop Relat Res 1998;353:231–7.
11. Mirra JM, Marder RA, Amstutz HC. The pathology of failed total joint arthroplasty. Clin Orthop Relat Res 1982;170:175–83.
12. Pinzur MS, Gil J, Belmares J. Treatment of osteomyelitis in Charcot foot with single-stage resection of infection, correction of deformity, and maintenance with ring fixation. Foot Ankle Int 2012;33:1069–74.
13. Mueller MJ, Diamond JE, Delitto A, et al. Insensitivity, limited joint mobility, and plantar ulcers in patients with diabetes mellitus. Phys Ther 1989;69:453–9.
14. Armstrong DG, Stapoole-Shea S, Nguyen H, et al. Lengthening of the Achilles tendon in diabetic patients who are at high risk for ulceration of the foot. J Bone Joint Surg Am 1999;81:535–8.
15. Mueller M, Sinacore DR, Hastings MK, et al. Effect of Achilles tendon lengthening on neuropathic plantar ulcers. A randomized clinical trial. J Bone Joint Surg Am 2003;85-A:1436–45.
16. Holstein P, Lohmann M, Bitsch M, et al. Achilles tendon lengthening, the panacea for plantar forefoot ulceration? Diabetes Metab Res Rev 2004;20(Suppl 1): S37–40.
17. Rong K, Li XC, Ge WT, et al. Comparison of the efficacy of three isolated gastrocnemius recession procedures in a cadaveric model of gastrocnemius tightness. Int Orthop 2016;40:417–23.
18. Firth GB, McMullan M, Chin T, et al. Lengthening of the gastrocnemius-soleus complex: an anatomical and biomechanical study in human cadavers. J Bone Joint Surg Am 2013;95:1489–96.
19. Sammarco VJ. Superconstructs in the treatment of Charcot foot deformity: plantar plating, locked plating, and axial screw fixation. Foot Ankle Clin 2009;14: 393–407.
20. Hruska KA, Teitelbaum SL. Renal osteodystrophy. N Engl J Med 1995;333: 166–74.

Circular External Fixation as a Primary or Adjunctive Therapy for the Podoplastic Approach of the Diabetic Charcot Foot

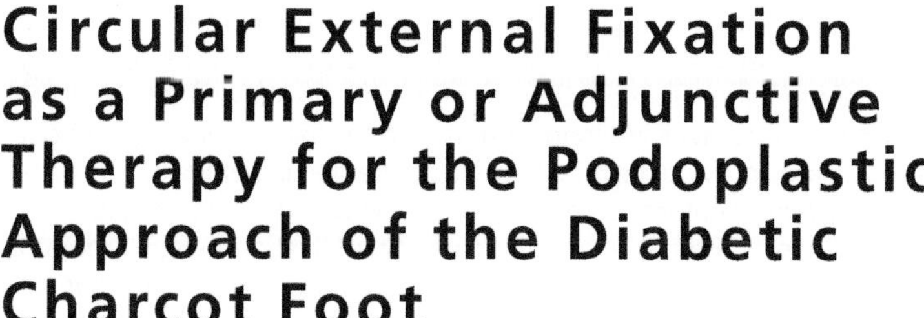

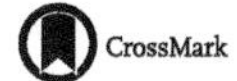

Daniel J. Short, DPM, Thomas Zgonis, DPM*

KEYWORDS

• External fixation • Diabetic Charcot foot • Charcot neuroarthropathy
• Podoplastic approach • Diabetic neuropathy • Plastic surgery

KEY POINTS

- External fixation can provide simultaneous compression, stabilization, and surgical offloading.
- Staged reconstruction is recommended in the ulcerated and/or infected diabetic Charcot foot.
- The podoplastic approach can achieve a combined skeletal and soft tissue reconstruction for surgical reconstruction of the diabetic Charcot foot.
- A multidisciplinary health care team that deals in the overall medical and surgical management of the diabetic patient is necessary for the patient's successful outcome.
- Close postoperative monitoring and management of the patient's medical comorbidities are vital throughout the recovery process.

Diabetic Charcot neuroarthropathy (DCN) foot and ankle deformities continue to be one of the most challenging clinical problems that face foot and ankle specialists. Conventional treatment options involve immobilization and local wound care modalities in order to achieve healing of wounds ranging from a variety of means to produce a healthy moist wound environment aimed at healing through secondary intention. Immobilization of the DCN lower extremity often involves limited or non-weight-bearing in a

Disclosure: The authors have nothing to disclose. T. Zgonis is the Consulting Editor for the *Clinics in Podiatric Medicine and Surgery*.
Reconstructive Foot and Ankle Surgery, Division of Podiatric Medicine and Surgery, Department of Orthopaedics, University of Texas Health Science Center San Antonio, 7703 Floyd Curl Drive, MSC 7776, San Antonio, TX 78229, USA
* Corresponding author.
E-mail address: zgonis@uthscsa.edu

Clin Podiatr Med Surg 34 (2017) 93–98
http://dx.doi.org/10.1016/j.cpm.2016.07.010
podiatric.theclinics.com

total contact cast; however, there is little evidence to support this treatment. The goal of DCN management is to achieve a stable, plantigrade, and braceable lower extremity, which is free from ulceration and infection. Several studies have shown that traditional methods of DCN management involving long-term accommodative nonsurgical treatments are unsuccessful at improving the quality of life of affected individuals.[1,2] In order to achieve the goals of management, surgery is often indicated in the unstable and symptomatic DCN. The use of internal, external, or combined fixation is usually dependent on the presence of a wound and/or osteomyelitis, anatomic location, vascular status, ambulation, medical comorbidities, and morbidity status. In certain cases, osseous exostectomies with or without plastic surgery closure and/or external fixation for surgical offloading might be indicated as the definitive procedures for the DCN.

CIRCULAR EXTERNAL FIXATION AS A PRIMARY TREATMENT FOR THE DIABETIC CHARCOT FOOT

Patients with DCN have poor bone quality and localized osteoporosis, as well as being poor immune hosts. Standard rigid internal fixation does not always lend itself to favorable osseous purchase in this population and has been shown to have decreased pull-out strength.[3] In addition, complete foot and/or ankle arthrodesis is not routinely achieved in the DCN, which over time with repetitive loading will lead to implant failure and breakage.

Ulceration caused by an underlying DCN deformity, infection, instability, and a non-plantigrade foot are several indications that may require surgical intervention. Location of fracture, nonunion, and deformity vary, and surgical reconstruction should be tailored to the individual patient. The first step in any reconstruction is thorough preoperative planning and evaluation of deformity. When deformity and instability are present, there is literature that shows these patients do progress toward ulceration.[4–7] A direct surgical approach including excision of the ulceration and/or infected bone is usually the preferred method of treatment because it allows access to the underling abnormality that needs to be corrected.

Osseous correction is achieved with exostectomy, osteotomy, and/or arthrodesis, whereas advanced deformities often require a combination of all 3. Once osseous correction is achieved intraoperatively, the osseous segments can be temporarily fixated with a Steinmann pin or pins; wounds are closed, and circular external fixation is applied and modified based on the surgical procedure performed. In a cadaveric model, it has been shown that the compression achieved through external fixation averaged 186% of the compression of screws alone.[8] Another advantage is that the compression can be increased postoperatively in a clinical or surgical setting when desired through manipulation of the external fixation system.

The beginning of external fixation begins proximally, in the distal tibia. A double tibial ring block is preferred for most of the DCN reconstructions because of the increased stability of the construct. Two tibial rings, connected by threaded rods, are placed to the distal tibia. Care must be taken to avoid the posterior ankle recess, which extends approximately 2 cm from the ankle joint, because wires within this area are technically intra-articular and could lead to septic joint. Smooth wires and/or half pins are then used to transfix the tibia and are mounted to the rings.

With the use of a midfoot ring, external fixation is able to correct for abduction/adduction of the midfoot, varus/valgus of the midfoot and/or hindfoot, and equinus. There are several options for connection of the midfoot ring to the tibial ring block, and the use of Ilizarov hinges allows for stable connection while applying compression and correcting the underlying deformity. In the setting of midfoot correction, further compression can be applied. The use of a midfoot ring completely offloads the entire foot and leg as it provides complete enclosure. The application of a kickstand provides additional offloading and elevates the limb, which allows drainage of the foot and protection of any advanced plastic procedure (**Fig. 1**).

THE PODOPLASTIC APPROACH FOR SURGICAL RECONSTRUCTION OF THE DIABETIC CHARCOT FOOT

In the presence of an open wound or osteomyelitis, DCN lower extremity reconstruction is best achieved by a combination of circular external fixation and plastic surgical closure (podoplastic approach). Circular external fixation is able to provide compression and stabilization across the prepared joint(s) for arthrodesis. In addition, it can

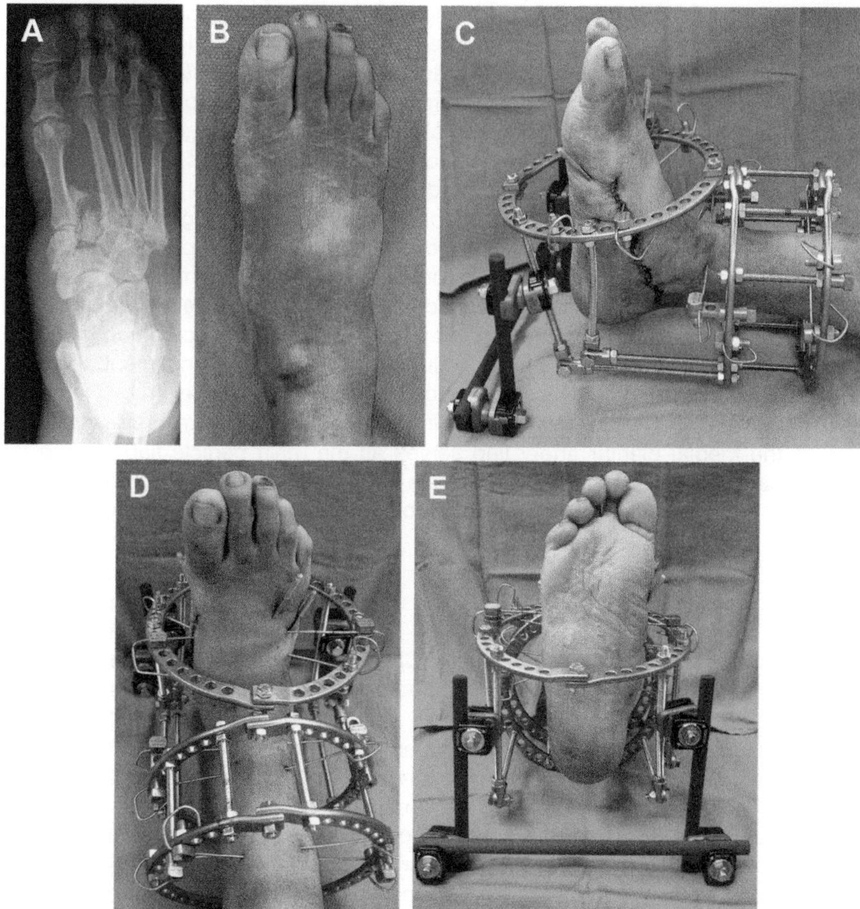

Fig. 1. Preoperative anteroposterior radiograph (*A*) and clinical picture (*B*) of a diabetic Charcot midfoot fracture-dislocation with joint instability. Utilization of circular external fixation as a primary surgical treatment of medial column arthrodesis (*C*), lateral column stabilization (*D*), and surgical offloading of the diabetic lower extremity (*E*). Please note the circular midfoot ring that allows for midfoot deformity correction (*C*, *D*) and additional kickstand apparatus for leg elevation and surgical offloading (*E*).

also correct any associated equinus deformities with the DCN. Open or percutaneous tendo-Achilles lengthening versus gastrocnemius recession may be necessary to assist in the overall osseous deformity correction and soft tissue reconstruction of the DCN. This type of circular external fixation is minimally invasive with the use of smooth wires compared with half pins. It also allows the simultaneous compression, stabilization, and correction of equinus that other constructs may be difficult to achieve. In addition, the use of smooth wires versus half pins has fewer complications in the diabetic population.[9]

Concomitant osteomyelitis and/or recurrent ulcerations require staged reconstruction in the DCN patient. Eradication of localized infection is paramount before the final procedure is determined. Circular external fixation becomes a great tool in the initial and final stages of reconstruction by providing stabilization, deformity correction, and surgically offloading major flap closure procedures. In addition, circular external fixation can also be used as an adjunctive procedure in assisting plastic surgical closure and equinus correction when dealing with chronic nonhealing wounds without osseous reconstruction. External fixation allows for direct wound visualization and easy access to wound dressing changes, assessment for flap closure viability, maintaining equinus correction, and providing immobilization of the foot to the lower extremity while surgically offloading the flap closure.

The circular external fixation construct for surgical offloading of the DCN in most cases is similar to the one used for arthrodesis procedures in the DCN patient. It is usually assembled by a 2-ring tibial block followed by a midfoot ring connected by Ilizarov hinges to assist in the equinus correction if needed. The application of a kickstand is paramount to assist in the podoplastic approach for the DCN. Dressing changes for flap viability are performed according to the flap closure technique, which may include a local, muscle, perforator, or pedicle closure. Most common local flap closure techniques for the DCN patient include the rotational advancement, transpositional, and rhomboid flaps. Muscle flap closure is commonly achieved by the use of the abductor hallucis, abductor digiti minimi, and flexor digitorum brevis muscles, whereas the medial plantar artery flap serves as the main pedicle flap closure for the DCN. Last, the reverse flow sural pedicle flap and perforator flaps based on the peroneal artery can serve for soft tissue reconstruction of major soft tissue defects of the DCN hindfoot and/or ankle (**Fig. 2**).

DISCUSSION

Acute or chronic plantar ulcerations in the DCN patient pose a serious clinical condition that may lead to soft tissue infection, osteomyelitis, septic arthritis, gas gangrene, lower extremity amputation, and systemic complications. Medical optimization, vascular assessment, and early surgical intervention when feasible are paramount to the patient's overall successful outcome. The multidisciplinary team includes health care providers from all services caring for the diabetic patient.

The podoplastic approach for surgical reconstruction of the DCN lower extremity provides a combined osseous and soft tissue reconstruction with stabilization and durable wound closure. In acute or chronic open wounds with DCN, staged reconstruction with skeletal and soft tissue reconstruction might be necessary to achieve wound closure and a stable deformity correction. The utilization of circular external fixation provides a multiplane correction while allowing the soft tissue reconstruction to be surgically offloaded and closely monitored throughout the postoperative period.[10] Frequent postoperative visits in a clinical setting can provide the opportunity for further external fixation adjustments if necessary.

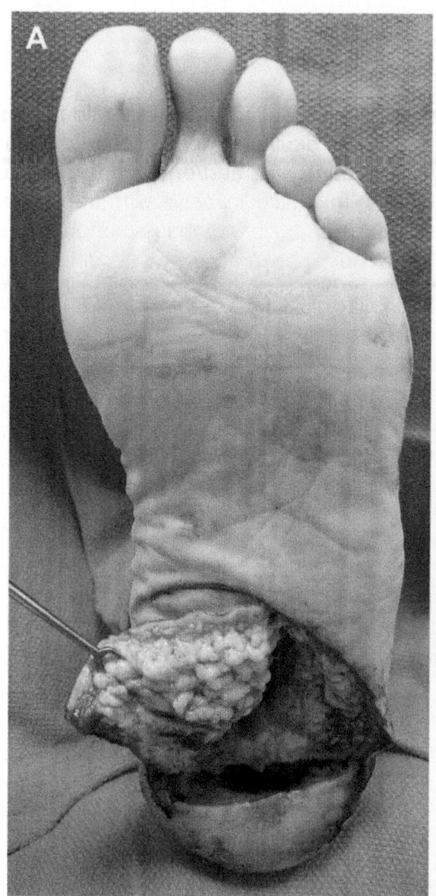

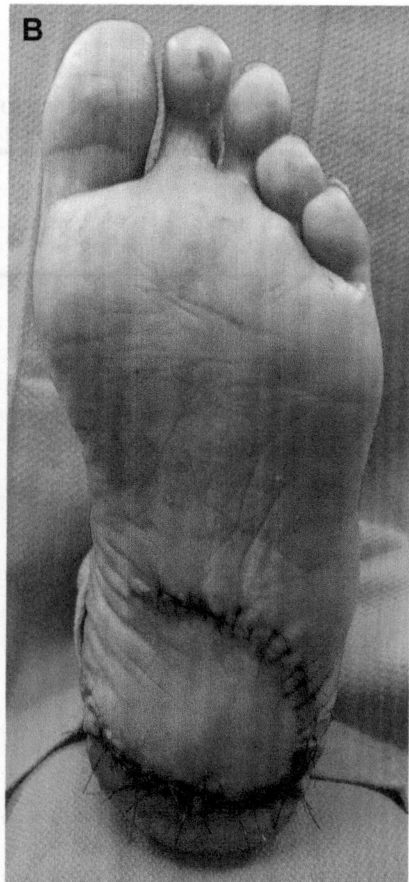

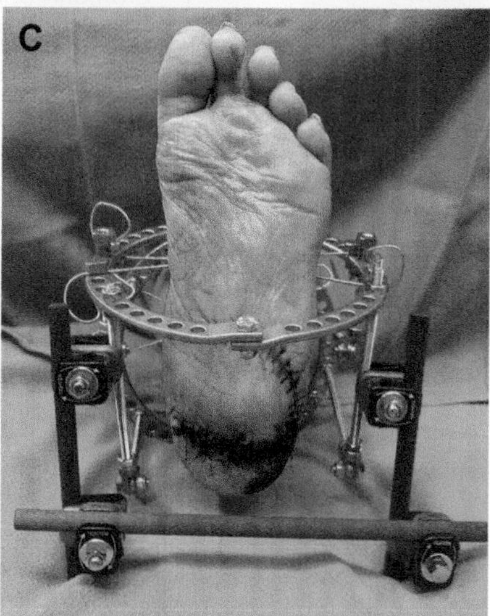

Fig. 2. Intraoperative clinical pictures (*A–C*) show the podoplastic surgical approach for reconstruction of the diabetic foot. (*A*) The raised local fasciocutaneous flap for insetting at the previously excised recipient wound in a triangular fashion (*B*). (*C*) Surgical offloading for the flap closure, stabilization of the foot to the lower extremity, and equinus correction if needed. This construct is similar when dealing with combined skeletal and soft tissue (podoplastic) reconstruction of the diabetic Charcot foot.

In summary, circular external fixation for surgical offloading of the diabetic foot as well as an adjunctive therapy for the podoplastic surgical approach of the DCN becomes a great surgical tool when dealing with the ulcerated and/or infected diabetic lower extremity.

REFERENCES

1. Dhawan V, Spratt KF, Pinzur MS, et al. Reliability of AOFAS diabetic foot questionnaire in Charcot arthropathy: stability, internal consistency, and measurable difference. Foot Ankle Int 2005;26:717–31.
2. Raspovic KM, Wukich DK. Self-reported quality of life in patients with diabetes: a comparison of patients with and without Charcot neuroarthropathy. Foot Ankle Int 2014;35:195–200.
3. Grant WP, Rubin LG, Pupp GR, et al. Mechanical testing of seven fixation methods for generation of compression across a midtarsal osteotomy: a comparison of internal and external fixation devices. J Foot Ankle Surg 2007;46:325–35.
4. Hastings MK, Johnson JE, Strube MJ, et al. Progression of foot deformity in Charcot neuropathic osteoarthropathy. J Bone Joint Surg Am 2013;95:1206–13.
5. Chantelau EA, Richter A. The acute diabetic Charcot foot managed on the basis of magnetic resonance imaging–a review of 71 cases. Swiss Med Wkly 2013;143: w13831.
6. Wukich DK, Raspovic KM, Hobizal KB, et al. Radiographic analysis of diabetic midfoot Charcot neuroarthropathy with and without midfoot ulceration. Foot Ankle Int 2014;35:1108–15.
7. Bevan WP, Tomlinson MP. Radiographic measures as a predictor of ulcer formation in diabetic Charcot midfoot. Foot Ankle Int 2008;29:568–73.
8. Latt LD, Glisson RR, Adams SB Jr, et al. Biomechanical comparison of external fixation and compression screws for transverse tarsal joint arthrodesis. Foot Ankle Int 2015;36:1235–42.
9. Jones CP, Youngblood CS, Waldrop N, et al. Tibial stress fracture secondary to half-pins in circular ring external fixation for Charcot foot. Foot Ankle Int 2014; 35:572–7.
10. Ramanujam CL, Facaros Z, Zgonis T. External fixation for surgical off-loading of diabetic soft tissue reconstruction. Clin Podiatr Med Surg 2011;28:211–6.

Index

Note: Page numbers of article titles are in **boldface** type.

Clin Podiatr Med Surg 34 (2017) 99–105
http://dx.doi.org/10.1016/S0891-8422(16)30115-X
0891-8422/17

F

G

H

I

J

L

M

N

O

P

R

S

T

U

V

W

Z

Printed and bound by CPI Group (UK) Ltd, Croydon, CR0 4YY
07/10/2024
01040500-0009